Kieran Cunningham is a Scottish climber and journalist who lived in Sondrio, Italy, a mountainous part of Lombardy which lies south of the Swiss border and about fifty miles from Lake Como. He lived there for six years, having arrived as a teacher and then switching to a full-time career as a climbing journalist, writing for the *Observer*, *Little India*, *Cool of the Wild* and *Moja Gear*, as well as editing the outdoors blog *My Open Country*.

CLIMBING THE WALLS

KIERAN CUNNINGHAM

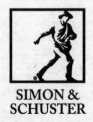

**SIMON &
SCHUSTER**

London · New York · Sydney · Toronto · New Delhi

First published in Great Britain by Simon & Schuster UK Ltd, 2021
This edition published in Great Britain by Simon & Schuster UK Ltd, 2022

1 3 5 7 9 10 8 6 4 2

Simon & Schuster UK Ltd
1st Floor
222 Gray's Inn Road
London WC1X 8HB

www.simonandschuster.co.uk
www.simonandschuster.com.au
www.simonandschuster.co.in

Simon & Schuster Australia, Sydney
Simon & Schuster India, New Delhi

A CIP catalogue record for this book
is available from the British Library

This book is a memoir. It reflects the author's present recollections of
experiences over time. Some names and characteristics have been changed to
protect the privacy of individuals and some dialogue has been recreated.

Paperback ISBN: 978-1-3985-0022-8
eBook ISBN: 978-1-3985-0021-1

Typeset in Bembo by M Rules
Printed in the UK by CPI Group (UK) Ltd, Croydon, CR0 4YY

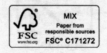

MIX
Paper from
responsible sources
FSC® C171272

For Bruno and Clementina

Lockdown −3 Days

We drive to Istanbul Airport in the late afternoon. Aiyla's checking her phone, reading me updates from the BBC, CNN, and *The Guardian*.

'I'm worried,' she says.

'You're always worried,' I say. 'I'm a Viking, remember? Ever hear of a Viking taken out by a microbe?'

She fakes a smile and throws herself into my shoulder, almost making me veer into a truck.

At the airport, no one appears to have heard of coronavirus. I see a couple of masks, a few guys washing their hands longer than usual in the toilets, but otherwise business as usual.

Aiyla waits at the gate as I head through security. Each time I turn around she's palming tears from her cheeks, her eyes drowning me with a wounded stare. I retrieve my backpack and jacket from the conveyor belt and head back down the line to console her.

'I'll be fine,' I tell her. 'I'll be back in a few weeks, virus-free. Promise.'

She grabs me by the cheeks and kisses me, the first time she's done so in public in Turkey.

I find my gate without having to look for the number, by following a group of fifteen Italians with Milanese accents. Their talk is of the virus. I hear the words 'bullshit', 'just a flu', and 'won't come to anything' in the twenty or so steps to the gate.

Onboard I have a whole row to myself and discover that the fifteen Milanese make up half of the plane's passengers.

I sleep two of the three hours to Milan Bergamo. When I wake, we're crossing the snow-capped peaks of the Bergamasque and Rhaetic Alps, the playground that has, these past six years, been my sanctuary, my safe haven from the world.

On our descent, the mountaintops look like clusters of French-tip icing on a cake. I make out the pyramidical outline of Corno Stella, the mountain where I almost died four years ago after crashing through a cornice while descending during a solo winter climb. I skidded for over 500 feet down the peak's north face, breaking my coccyx and three ribs on the way, and only avoided breaking the rest of myself by arresting my fall with my ice axe just a few yards above a 100-foot cliff. It took me nine hours to crawl back to my car and another two to negotiate the three-mile drive down the bumpy forest track to the valley floor and then to the hospital in Sondrio. For the next three months I hobbled around on crutches carrying a rubber swim-ring decorated with Smurfs as a cushion, much to the delight of my colleagues, students, friends and my fellow townspeople. It would be another nine months or so before I regained full fitness, but within a few days of the accident, the 'never again' I'd repeatedly muttered on the shuffle off the mountain on all fours had already been forgotten and I was itching to get back up there – just as I am now, after only ten days in Istanbul.

The airport in Bergamo is deserted. I check my watch to see if there's time to make the 7.20 p.m. train home and break into a jog after collecting my bags, but there's a line of people before customs. At its front, a trio of suited medics are taking the temperatures of the bemused travellers. One of the more bemused, a man in his fifties waving his passport, is firing a volley of invective over the heads of the crowd. An armed guard stops him when he attempts to skip past the doctors.

I miss the 7.20 by two minutes and wait at the station with a young Polish guy trying to get to Switzerland. We're the only two passengers on the three platforms. A cleaner is silently emptying bins.

On the 8.20 train, I have the carriage to myself. After arriving in Sondrio just before eleven, I haul my luggage through the cobbled streets, passing the bar where any other Friday night I'd find half a dozen friends standing outside drinking spritz and smoking. The bar is empty.

Lockdown −2 Days

I wake to my phone ringing: Matteo, my climbing partner. The training course he's been scheduled to attend has been called off as a precaution and he wants to go climbing.

We meet three more friends – Franco, Sasso, and Lucia – at one of our local crags, a 40-metre bluff of gneiss on a wooded slope above the apple orchards and vineyards of the village of Ponte, a few miles down the Valtellina valley from Sondrio. Between climbs the only talk is of the virus – preventative measures, the ten villages to the west on lockdown, the rising death toll, the outlook. It will come to nothing, they assure me.

'Nothing comes up this valley,' says Matteo. 'Not even tourists. Shit, not even the Romans. We'll be fine.'

As we're leaving the crag in the late afternoon, a farmer

pulls up on the cobbled road where we've parked and emerges in a mask from his three-wheeler van. He gives us a wide berth while making his way to the stone-built hut, outside which three goats have trotted over to greet him. Once past, he stops and calls after us.

'It's no good climbing in times like these. Your fun could be the death of someone!'

'He's right, you know,' says Lucia in the car. 'We shouldn't have been there.'

We go for dinner with Lucia's brother, Michele, his girl-friend, Simona, and their friend Mirko in Tirano, a town 15 miles east of Sondrio. I haven't seen them for at least a month but the usually obligatory *baci* (the kissing-on-cheeks upon which Italians insist) and hugs are replaced by elbow-bumps and awkward greetings at a one-metre remove.

We choose a bar in the town centre for a pre-dinner *aperitivo*. When we arrive, the solitary barman looks up accusingly from his phone. The place is playing music too upbeat for the mood. We're the only customers apart from a man with a dog snoozing at his feet at the bar and a pair of giggling teenagers in the corner.

'So, what's gonna happen with you and Aiyla now they're blocking flights out of Italy?' Simona asks when we sit at our table.

We talked about it on the phone that morning. Turkish authorities have suspended all flights to and from Italy until 10 April, meaning the trip I've planned for the end of the month will have to be postponed.

'I don't know. Looks like we'll just have to wait until it's over. Or meet at my parents' place in Scotland.'

'Who says Scotland will be safe?'

'It doesn't have any cases yet. Or very few, at least.'

'It isn't going to be over for a while. You know that, right?' says Lucia.

'We'll see,' I say. 'It's not like—'

'All this,' interrupts Mirko, 'because those fucking Chinese wanna eat *bat* for dinner. What's wrong with rice, or pasta, or fish, or ham, or pizza?'

'Easy there, Signor Trump,' says Simona, smiling, but her face flushes. 'What's the difference between a bat and a pig?' She nods towards the plate of skewered cubes of ham and cheese on our table. 'They're both animals.'

'Yeah, but . . .'

'But nothing. It's just so fucking twenty-first century to use food as racism. I'm sick of it.'

'It ain't racism, Simo, it's just a fact. They have uncivilised habits and the rest of us are paying for it.'

'How about the other facts? Like, that just about every Chinese family in our valley has been physically or verbally abused since this all started. They've had to close their shops and restaurants because nobody goes there any more. Some are leaving. At work the other day, a Korean lady came in with a sprained ankle and I was the only nurse who'd go near her. Is that a good showing of civilisation? You think the Chinese are turning away Italians and spitting on them in their subways?'

The pizza place we move on to seems surprisingly busy until we learn it's the only one still open. Mid-meal, Lucia, who works at a logistics plant over the border in Switzerland, checks her phone and discovers the government is in talks to declare all of our region, Lombardy, a red zone.

Lockdown -1 Day

Five of us cram into the car for a trip up the neighbouring valley of Valmalenco.

'Shit,' says Matteo, squeezing in beside me. 'They're advising one metre of distance between each person, but your fat Scottish ass is leaving me less than a millimetre!'

Overnight the local authorities have recommended the closure of all bars, restaurants, cinemas, museums and all ski and sports facilities in the valley. As yet, though, nobody has suggested any restriction on mountaineering or ski-mountaineering. We may be flouting the guidelines on *distanziamento fisico* (social distancing) that have just been announced by the *Ministero della Salute* (Ministry of Health), but up here the whole thing still seems too remote to make anyone feel overly uneasy about being in such close proximity to others.

The traffic on the tortuous series of switchbacks that climb from the centre of Sondrio towards the Valmalenco valley is slightly lighter than usual, but not much. We're in a line of four or five cars, all with loaded ski racks, and before reaching the turn-off for Valmalenco pass at least a dozen cars and a handful of *ape* vans – the three-wheeled, rickshaw-style vehicles favoured by local farmers and vintners – descending into the town. Ahead, the grey-and-white heads of the Bernina Range's Roseg, Tremoggia and Gemelli peaks are yellowing in the first light.

Turning off outside the village of Lanzada, we catch sight of our day's objective – Pizzo Scalino, a 3,323-metre pyramid of ice and rock dubbed 'Il Cervino della Valmalenco' ('The Matterhorn of Valmalenco').

The car park is in a snowy bowl at 2,000 metres, and the

number of cars there suggests we aren't the only ones who've thought of getting around the ban by heading to the mountains.

The release is palpable as we ascend the mountain's lower flanks. I couldn't be feeling further from the panic and claustrophobia that has enveloped the valley since I returned from Istanbul.

But by the time we reach the first pass, Lucia has received a text message from her boyfriend telling her there's talk of closing the border that evening. She lives near Lake Lugano in Switzerland, just across the border and about two hours' drive from Sondrio. Closing the border would prevent her returning home and making it to work tomorrow.

We turn around and ski down to a rustic *agriturismo* serving goat's cheese and plates of polenta for a late lunch. When we arrive, the news channels are already awash with conflicting information about border controls and who will be able to travel to and from work outside the valley.

We sit outside on deckchairs in the snow in the warm afternoon sun. Spring is coming. A mountain guide I've met on previous climbing trips appears with a client. He sticks out his hand before pulling it back and offering me an elbow.

'So,' he says, 'it's true after all. Mountaineers are the only free ones.'

'It looks like it . . .'

'It must be a year since I last saw you. Still living here?'

'Yeah,' I say. 'It's home now.'

'Still teaching?'

'Nah. I gave it up. I realised I could get by doing some freelance journalism online. It gives me more time to do this.'

'Wait,' he says, tugging a lock of his long curls behind his ear. 'So you're free to work and live anywhere you like, and you choose to be here?'

'It's paradise here. My girlfriend lives in Turkey. If I can convince her to move over, I'll never leave.'

That night the news comes that the lockdown will be extended to all of Italy until 3 April, and all travel to, from and within Lombardy will be banned. The only permitted movement will be to workplaces, or for 'essential' visits to the doctor or supermarket.

Lockdown Day 1

Half-asleep, I imagine myself in Istanbul, hearing the morning *azan* from the mosque.

Soon I realise the voice is Italian, issuing from a megaphone somewhere in the street below my apartment:

'Ladies and gentlemen, in accordance with the latest restrictions issued by the Ministry of Health, we advise all citizens to remain at home. Those with auto-certification or permission to be at large are reminded to remain at least one metre from others at all times.'

The refrain continues throughout the morning.

Over breakfast I check my food supplies and find I have enough for a few days. My phone pings multiple times while I read through the news online. Most of the messages are jokes, attempts to make light of things despite the unnerving figures of deaths and cases of infection, which are rising steadily each day; others are short video clips showing thousands of people fleeing Lombardy for the south of the country in the hours before the lockdown took effect.

Soon, my social media feeds are awash with communications

from the national mountaineering organisation, the Club Alpino Italiano, announcing that all mountaineering and climbing activity is prohibited with immediate effect.

For the first time, the potential impact hits home. I work freelance as a journalist. Each weekday I rise at 4 a.m. and finish work by lunchtime, then take to the mountains until dusk, spending an average of three hours outside climbing, ski-mountaineering, ice-climbing, bouldering or just hiking in the woods above the town. In really bad weather, I drive to an indoor climbing wall in Valmalenco to put in my daily quota of climbs. As a sufferer of Bipolar 1, this is my coping strategy, the only regime that forestalls the volatile mental states I've experienced in every other job I've had, or when deprived of my fill of fresh mountain air and exercise. It's why I moved to these mountains six years ago and, over the years, is something that I've learned is every bit as vital to dealing with the symptoms of Bipolar 1 as my medication. Today's message states that all climbing crags and gyms will be closed until further notice. Ski-mountaineering is also prohibited. Anyone caught in a vehicle with skis will be handed an on-the-spot fine of €206. I shuffle to the bathroom in my slippers and check my meds. My mum sends me my pills every month, but I have no idea if the post will continue running and don't want her anywhere near a post office even if it does. I find three boxes. One is empty, but the other two have thirty-three pills between them – enough to see me through the lockdown period barring any extensions. I try not to panic. Things will get better soon. Normal life will resume.

My daily meditation of twenty-five minutes runs an hour longer than usual. For the first time that I can remember since childhood, there is a surfeit of time.

In lieu of my morning jog I hop on the cross trainer left behind by my apartment's previous occupant and kill another hour.

My mother calls, as she has done at least three times daily since the news broke of Italy's first cases.

'Don't worry, Ma. Even if I get it, I'm apparently too young and healthy to come to real harm.'

Her sharp intake of breath tells me to change tack.

'It's fine, Ma. I'm staying at home. I have everything I need and I'm ready to sit it out as long as need be.'

'What about your medication?'

'I mean *everything*, Ma. Gloves, masks, food, meds, reading material – everything. When the kilo of heroin I ordered online arrives this afternoon, I'll be all set.'

Just a day into the official quarantine and less than a week after the red-zone declaration, I already feel like a lockdown veteran compared to friends and family scattered across the globe. The British response appears woefully inept – to the point of criminality. And the thought of the fate and well-being of my parents – both fast approaching seventy and potentially 'high-risk' – being in the hands of the fruitcakes who masterminded Brexit, and who seem hell-bent on depriving us of universal healthcare, put knots in my gut.

Here in Italy, the streets are empty, workplaces have shut down, trains have stopped running; police teams are patrolling the streets and fining those who've gone A(from home)WOL, supermarkets are enforcing a strict one-in/one-out policy; the government is releasing almost hourly communiqués on nationwide developments, financial relief for local businesses and homeowners, recommended safety measures and updated policies. Back home, people are panic-buying toilet paper.

Next on the line is Aiyla. Turkey has yet to register its first case. She suspects that the government is attempting to keep it under wraps to avoid the economy taking a hit.

Aiyla and I met in St Andrews two summers ago when I was home visiting my parents and she was over on a staff exchange at the university. We went on a couple of dates and promised to keep in touch when she returned to Turkey. Since then, we've video-called every day and alternated monthly trips to Sondrio and Istanbul, but it's only been in the last few months that we've started talking seriously about building a life together, whether in Turkey, Scotland or Italy. On this last visit, we started discussing when, and how, to break the news about our relationship to her conservative Muslim family. Now it looks like we'll be forced to wait.

When she hangs up, I call it a day and turn in for the night, hoping tomorrow will be brighter. As I make my way to the bathroom to brush my teeth, I glance at the clock on the kitchen wall.

It's 8.30 p.m.

Lockdown Day 2

My morning's work is interrupted by an onslaught of concerned messages from friends in the US, Germany, the UK, Portugal, India and even Sicily. I can't help but feel uneasy. All this, I know, is coming their way.

In many ways I feel fortunate to live in such a remote part of the globe. And a remote part within that remote part, at that. I live on the lower floor of a two-storey house situated in a small vineyard above the town, at least half a mile from the nearest bar or supermarket, or any place where people are likely to congregate in numbers. The only person I'm likely to see without venturing into the town is my landlady, Giuseppina, the 90-year-old widow who lives on the floor above and is prone to sending down care packages of coffee and cake, cured meats and other edibles on an almost daily basis.

In the six years I've been here, Giuseppina has come to treat me like family: inviting me up for lunch or dinner with her grandchildren once a week, insisting that I leave her a note whenever I go to the mountains alone, and calling to check up on me when I'm away visiting Aiyla, my parents or my sister in Brooklyn. Since the death two years ago of her husband, Domenico, Giuseppina's health has suffered, robbing her of some of her former vitality and infectious cheerfulness. Nevertheless, her face is permanently on the verge of a smile and every morning she appears in the garden at nine, her chin-length bob neatly brushed, and dressed immaculately in ankle-length skirts or slacks with floral blouses and woollen cardigans, and a pair of leather Mary Janes on her feet. She carefully inspects her flowers then either waves to me at my window or knocks on my door to tell me off if she hasn't heard from me in a few days.

A glorious day is brewing. So glorious that I'm forced to bring down my shutters to avoid anger at missing out on an afternoon of climbing.

More pings on my phone convince me to turn it off while I work.

Around noon I peel the last sheet of toilet paper off the roll and find no replacement in the cabinet beneath the sink. I scour my apartment for any other form of tissue paper and dig up one lonesome paper napkin in my cutlery drawer and an antiquated, mangled tissue that may or may not have been used. I return to the bathroom, sure that there must be a roll hidden somewhere, but no . . .

While unfolding the napkin, my eyes land on the fitting that has remained disused throughout my six-year tenancy: the *bidet*.

I place the napkin by the sink. A twist of the tap on the bidet brings forth a gush of water. It's far too cold so I wait until the temperature has risen, but then notice the angle of the flow appears . . . well, logistically suboptimal. For the first time in those half-dozen years, I spy a nozzle on the tap's tip. A slight recalibration redirects the gushing flow first onto my shirt and then across the floor. I switch it off. When I turn it back on again after a readjustment, the flow is again directed safely inside the bowl but appears only to heat up when at full power, thus ruling out the possibility of angling the nozzle towards its desired target before that target is *in situ*.

I hover over the seatless bowl until my clenched buttocks make contact with the cold ceramic surface. On first impact, the feel of the even-colder water is among the most discomfiting sensations I can claim to have experienced, but as I increase the flow by reaching behind me to turn the tap, the initial unpleasantness dissolves in the increasingly tepid gush. After a further five minutes with the balmy jet of water buffeting my posterior, I am converted.

I work the rest of the afternoon. At dinner time, I applaud myself for coping with my second day of quarantine. Beyond my success with the bidet, I've completed a full day of work, done laundry in my breaks, emptied the dishwasher, and retained a degree of calm and stoic acceptance that I could not have anticipated.

But then I remember I'm at the epicentre of one of the world's most serious health crises in decades and that there are people who may be wondering about my welfare.

The key to surviving, I think – as I restart my phone after the longest break it has known, to send out an 'alive and well' to my family and Aiyla – would not only be self-isolation from the microbial aggressors at large and their human hosts, but also self-isolation from the ever-maddening and increasingly unhinged response of those they threaten.

Fear is a virus itself.

Lockdown Day 3

The daily death tolls are rising. Yesterday, they breached 100 for the first time. Things are going to get a whole lot worse.

I take my laptop out onto my small terrace to work in the sun. At one point I hear the lock on the door upstairs and scramble to get inside; if reports are to be believed, Giuseppina's age and health issues put her at serious risk.

But before I can fully retreat inside my apartment, I hear her call my name.

'I don't want to risk infecting you,' I shout through a slim opening in the terrace door.

'Let me see you, lad,' she replies. My door is directly beneath Giuseppina's and my terrace under the staircase that leads from the front gate up to the landing outside her door. I can hear that she's still at the top of her stairs, more than three metres from my terrace. When I emerge again, I find her leaning over the banister, dressed in her pyjamas and bathrobe.

'*Ciao!*' she cries, giggling. 'How is it going down there?'

'It's going well. As well as it can, I mean. I'm working.'

'It will pass. You shouldn't be stressing yourself with so much work in times like these. Rest a little.'

'Maybe I will.'

'Look. Have you seen the flowers?'

The cherry trees on the bottom tier of the garden have burst into flower – hundreds of pink flutes reaching skyward like Roman candles against the backdrop of the snowy peaks in the distance. I hadn't noticed until now.

'Yes,' she says. 'All this will pass. When I was a girl the young men went to war. We hid in the underground tunnels when the bombs came, with our families – down there, on Via Scarpatetti. Now we just have to stay at home. It's no great imposition, is it? All these things pass. Take care of yourself, Kieran. And eat more. If you need anything, let me know.'

Once she has gone back inside, I turn on my phone to call my mother. It erupts with notifications. I ignore all bar a WhatsApp group chat with close friends, in which I find a message from Simona, who's been placed in 14-day isolation after her sister tested positive. She warns us that she may have become infected before our dinner and day's skiing together at the weekend. Reports claim the virus can remain in the system for as long as ten days without the appearance of symptoms, so she warns us all to be vigilant.

That night I become my own watchman. A small cough after dinner sees me on Google researching symptoms and a more precise definition of what type of cough to fear.

In bed I lie awake. Am I sweating? No, not sweating. Breathless? Nah. Cold? Maybe a little, but I've left the window open. I get up and Google the symptoms again just to be sure.

Lockdown Day 4

Rain today.

I work through the morning. For variety, I've decided to shift my work station around the apartment. The house stands on a slope not far below the highest point in the town. From my kitchen, I have a view across the top of the largest section of the vineyard, on the west side of the house, to Castel Masegra, a fourteenth-century castle squatting on a nearby hill above the town, just 250 metres or so away. My bedroom window faces south, down the length of the vineyard to the top of Via Scarpatetti, at the heart of the old town, and over the tiled roof-tops and cobbled streets to the clock tower in the town centre and the *Alpi Orobie* – the Bergamasque Alps – on the other side of the valley. From my living room, I can look west towards the lower valley and the villages of Caiolo, Cedrasco and Colorina at the foot of the Orobie, and east over our neighbour's garden, as far as the village of Piateda, four miles away, directly below the fang-like summit of Punta di Santo Stefano. Today, I choose the bedroom.

In the streets below there is no movement, no sound, no sign of life whatsoever.

Between spells at the computer I phone my sister, mother and father to update them. I also clear out my cupboard of climbing gear, polish every wooden surface in the apartment and make a start on a small alp of ironing that's become an almost permanent fixture. While tidying the cupboard, I shake out a handful of sand from the running shoes I'd taken home on my last visit to Scotland. My parents live in a small village, Lundin Links, on the east coast. Beneath the village, two beaches extend for miles in either direction. My imagination carries me back there momentarily as I'm cleaning up the sand. I wonder how long it might be before I see the place again.

After completing my work for the day, I'm amazed to discover it's not even 2 p.m. and wonder what I usually do with the hours. I message my friends in the valley to check up on them and then sit for another half-hour of meditation. The barking of my neighbour's dog in his enclosure is a welcome interruption to the silence. Next, I hear sirens. One has barely faded when another begins to sound from the opposite direction.

I return to doing chores and find my supply of protein and vegetables is precariously low. The inevitable can no longer be avoided. I pull five biodegradable shopping bags from a drawer and stuff a mask and tube of hand sanitiser in my pocket along with a €100 note.

On the drive to the supermarket I pass Carabinieri and Guardia di Finanza and *polizia locale*, three different divisions of local policing authorities. I'm surprised that none of them stops me. Each day my Facebook feed fills with tales of those who've been less fortunate and been handed fines for being outside their homes without the requisite documentation (or dog).

There are more cars in the supermarket car park than I expected – maybe twelve in total. Then again, grocery shopping is one of only four permissible activities (along with dog-walking, giving kids fresh air and trips to the pharmacy), and already I could forgive anyone who has chosen to exaggerate their need for provisions to justify breaking the monotony.

I put on my mask before leaving the car and remind myself of the essentials: no basket, no trolley, touch as little as possible, stay well clear of everyone.

Inside, I spot eight heads above the rows of goods. In the first aisle, I find myself caught, with a masked fellow shopper, in that soon-to-be-familiar shuffle where two people heading in opposing directions attempt to get out of each other's way, only to get in it instead. Not a good start. Eventually I skip past and begin loading my bags with the items on my mental shopping list – coffee, flour, chicken, milk, eggs, tinned tuna, hand soap, salad, biscuits, detergent, more biscuits, more chicken, a few frozen meals and a few handfuls of fruit. I'm surprised to find the shelves fully stocked. Online pictures from the UK this morning showed ransacked supermarkets and shelves empty of pasta, rice, toilet paper and soap. Here nothing is out of stock except hand sanitiser. As I hit the TP section, I decide to pass, mentally claiming a small victory over the world.

The masked-to-unmasked ratio is a straight 50:50, but everyone is steering clear of everyone else to the tune of one metre or more, and at the checkout area there are taped lines on the floor at 1.5-metre intervals. Waiting in line, I spot a man of around sixty in a hurry, rounding the aisles as though improvising a racetrack. He reappears at my shoulder a minute or so later and coughs, forcibly. I imagine millions of little coronavirus missiles swarming in a dense cloud before me and shift lane, consoling myself with the guilty thought that if my assailant is in fact infected, then his age and all relevant statistics to date dictate that he will be the most likely of the two of us to die.

Outside I load the car before taking off the plastic gloves supplied at the entrance and dropping them in a litter bin. Already I understand that the risk of contamination posed by the trip is far from over. I rub my hands down with sanitiser and run an alcohol-rich wet-wipe over my face.

In town, at the first roundabout, I'm stopped by the Carabinieri. The unmasked officer asks me where I'm going and where I've been. Before I've finished explaining he waves me through.

Back home I place my bags of shopping in the bathtub and wash my hands. I remove all non-packaged items from the bags and wash them in the kitchen sink before placing them away in the fridge or cupboards. I discard the bags, rewash my hands, then line up all of the packaged items in the bath. I skoosh shower gel over the top of them like syrup on pancakes, then rinse them off with the shower hose and leave them to dry. Next, I wipe down everything I've touched since arriving home with antibacterial soap and a cloth, and remind myself to buy fourteen days' worth of food next time instead of seven.

Lockdown Day 5

Sirens again. Every quarter of an hour or so. Where are they going?

While drinking my morning coffee, I call my mother, who updates me on her revised MO.

'I'll only go for one coffee per day. And not to the hotel or to the busy cafés in St Andrews; just the farmhouse one. The tables there are well spread-out and they're always very clean.'

'Ma . . .'

'And no more shopping. Only for emergencies and

necessities. I already have all the boxes of pasta and toilet paper from when they were warning us about Brexit, but now I'm filling your sister's room with more things. I mean, who knows how long this will last . . .'

'Ma, it's great you're planning to scale down your, eh . . . stuff. But I really think you should be taking things a little more seriously. You and Dad both have what could be considered "pre-existing conditions", after all.'

'But I am taking it seriously. Do you think I should stop going to the gym? Boris Johnson was on yesterday: he says we're not to panic.'

That morning I'd read the British premier's containment plan and was horrified to discover very little in the way of containment.

'I think you should be panicking just a little more, Ma. And no, no more gym. And tell Dad to stop going to the climbing wall. And maybe try having coffee at home. Walk along the beach. Take the dog for walks in the woods. Every interaction is a potential life-or-death situation – remember that. And not just for you – for everyone else you or they come into contact with afterwards.'

I call my sister, Cath. She works as an editor for a commercial property magazine in New York City and lives with her dachshund, Vincenzo, in a little apartment between Sunset Park and Park Slope in Brooklyn. We normally speak every other day, but she's just back from a holiday in Hawaii with her boyfriend and has been busy. New York busy is very different to Sondrio busy, keeping her in her office from 7 or 8 a.m. until 9 p.m., often for weeks on end. Things there seem to be escalating and she travels to work every day on the subway. I can't imagine a worse place to be. Her employers haven't yet okayed the work-from-home policy that their staff have petitioned for and her edginess is apparent. It seems a bit soon, but we agree to cancel my planned visit in May.

That night my head is ringing from twelve hours at my computer and breaks spent placating worried friends and family members on the phone. I sit at the window, slumped so low in my chair that I can only see the mountains across the valley. At that angle, the world is as it was three weeks ago, unsullied by the stain steadily expanding into its every corner. *If only I could be up there now*, I think, but have to nip the reverie in the bud before I let myself get carried away

I change into gym clothes, planning to put in an hour or so on the cross trainer. I didn't sleep well last night. It's the lack of activity, the lack of stimulus, the drowsy lethargy that's the defining feature of each day. I've barely started on the cross trainer when I have a change of heart. Instead, I change into trousers and walking shoes, and slip out of the apartment. It's dark, and the cool air is a balm on my skin. My lungs rejoice. I look up and down the street for anyone who might object to my breakout, but see no one.

I head uphill, passing the dozen or so houses that lie between my apartment and the huge expanse of vineyards that rises above the town. I reach the vineyards without incident or encounter. A sliver of guilt accompanies me each step of the way, but the chances of bumping into anyone are slim.

Balloon-like clouds, impossibly white, play in the light of a buttery, almost full moon. The snowy peaks sparkle across the valley. As part of my effort to stay sane as a work-from-home freelancer, I've walked through these vines hundreds of times, setting off in all weathers to stretch my legs and air my lungs between stints on my laptop. Never have they seemed more beautiful.

On the way back down the slope, the trail forks multiple times between the drystone walls that divide the vineyards of different owners. At one juncture I'm surprised by a black mass that appears in the corner of my eye. The black mass appears to be surprised by me, too, uttering a profanity and apology in a single breath before hurrying on down the trail.

I video-call Aiyla before bed.

'We're only five days in and I'm already dreaming about the mountains,' I tell her.

'For a moment there, I thought you were going to tell me you were dreaming about me. You realise this qualifies as an obsession, right?'

Yes, but explaining it to non-climbers is never easy. How do you persuade someone of the beauty and merit in something that's so patently dangerous, arduous and almost invariably painful? My ice-climbing partner, Luigi, never misses an opportunity to remind me that '*l'alpinismo è sofferenza*' ('mountaineering is suffering'). He works as an insurance broker in Sondrio's town centre and for the past five winters has taken it upon himself to show me all the big ice-climbs in the area. When we climb together, our friends call us '*Le Torri Gemelle*' ('The Twin Towers') on account of us both being 6ft 3ins tall, roughly half a foot above the group average. He's fifty-six years old and has been climbing for over forty years, but still has the enthusiasm of a newbie.

'People don't understand,' he says, 'that suffering can be a good thing. How can you know A without knowing Z, eh? My ex-wife used to take offence that I'd choose all you smelly bastards and ice and rock over her. She was a lawyer. Soulless. I should never have married a woman who doesn't climb, and you shouldn't either, *giovane*.'

A month after I met Luigi, he came to talk to me one afternoon while I was climbing at our local crag, Sassella; he'd just finished work and was dressed in shirt, tie, slacks and brogues. He scrambled up the rocky approach to the climbing area, clutching his jacket in one hand.

'What are you doing this weekend, Highlander?' he asked, loosening his tie.

'Nothing. Why?'

'Pack your rucksack. We're doing the Biancograt.'

The Biancograt is an epic three-day route that begins in the Engadin valley in Switzerland, not far from St Moritz, about an hour and a half away from Sondrio. It climbs a series of glaciers and fin-like rock-and-snow ridges to the summit of Piz Bernina (4,040 metres), the highest mountain in the eastern Alps, before descending back into Italy via two more glaciers and a long hike that ends in the upper Valmalenco valley, less than a mile from where Lucia, Simona, Matteo, Sasso and I set off on our skis the day before lockdown. It's considered one of the classic climbs in the Alps and was one I'd had on my tick-list for years.

We left Sondrio at four in the morning on the Saturday. We were joined by Luigi's friend and boss, David, a fortysomething sport climber I'd first met one day at Sassella, when I'd watched him spend his lunchbreak free-soloing a trio of routes that I'd struggle to take on even with ropes. We left the car in the village of Pontresina, five miles from St Moritz, and hiked up the long, forested Roseg Valley before turning off to climb the steep banks of glacial moraine along the flanks of the Tschierva Glacier up to a *rifugio* (mountain hut) at 2,600 metres. We spent the night in the hut and set off at one the next morning with head torches and crampons, crossing the foot of the glacier on the way to a narrow col just below the three-kilometre ridge that constitutes the Biancograt proper. The headlamps of the twenty or so other mountaineers and guides we'd shared the hut with bored tunnels of light into the inky darkness above and below us on the glacier and the only sound was the scratching of crampons on ice and rock.

The glacier steepened and narrowed below the col, bottle-necking between a rocky bluff on the flanks of Piz Morteratsch to the left and, to the right, the towering cliff face we'd be climbing over to reach the start of the long summit ridge. We stopped for a drink and to let the team in front get ahead of us so we could avoid placing ourselves in the fall-line of any rocks they might knock down onto the route once on the cliff above. While waiting, we heard the crunch of crampons in the darkness to our left, at least 20 metres from the route in an area pocked with crevasses. Then, a voice.

'*Scheisse!*' it said.

We aimed our headlamps in the direction of the voice and saw a figure hunched over, on one knee, on a small island of snow between two large crevasses.

'*Ma che cazzo sta facendo?*' said David. *What the fuck is he doing?*

'A suicide,' said Luigi.

I couldn't believe what I was seeing. The slope we were on

was at an angle of at least 55 degrees, iced over and riddled with deep crevasses, yet the man appeared to be unroped, without a partner or ice axe, and unable to stay on his feet.

'Excuse me, *signor*,' Luigi called to the man. 'Do you need help?'

'*Ich spreche kein Italien!*'

The man tried to take a step towards us but slipped onto his side.

'Wait!' shouted Luigi.

We built an anchor in the snow with an ice screw and ice axe, and I belayed Luigi while he went over to fetch the German. When they returned, we saw that the man was old, maybe in his seventies. He was wearing rustic crampons with spikes worn to their last centimetre, and carrying a wooden-shafted snow pick that was no more than a foot and a half long. I'd only ever seen them in museums.

Luigi, who speaks a few words of German, asked the man a few questions and learned that he was alone. He'd joined a team who'd left the hut at midnight but they'd abandoned him at the foot of the glacier because he was too slow. They'd told him to go back to the hut, but he'd thought he might be able to do the route alone.

'Crazy old bastard,' said David, 'and irresponsible too. Now he's our responsibility. What the fuck are we supposed to do with a 100-year-old German dressed for *Carnavale*? If we send him back, he'll end up in a crevasse.'

'Let's take him with us,' said Luigi.

'What? He doesn't even have a harness!' David replied. 'How the hell do you rope up with someone who doesn't have a harness?'

'I'll make one for him,' Luigi said. 'If we take him back to the hut, we'll lose three or four hours. Anyway, there are four of us now, and it's always better to work in teams of two. We have two ropes so, David, you go with the Scotsman and I'll take the German.'

Luigi fashioned a harness from a large sling and buddied up with the German.

In the next hour, we learned that the German's name was Anders and he was seventy years old. He'd chosen to do the Biancograt because he'd spent the spring and early part of the summer visiting his sister in a hospice in Graubünden and hadn't seen the mountains in months. He'd always dreamed of climbing Piz Bernina, he said, and his usual companion had died last year.

We also learned that Anders had never belayed a partner or abseiled before. On his first attempt at belaying, he dropped Luigi five metres down an ice gulley before finally stopping the rope. On a short abseil down the side of a thumb-like *gendarme* on the ridge, he lost his grip on the rope while still three metres from the rocky ledge where I was waiting for him with David. He landed with one foot on my hand, his crampon slicing open my glove and leaving a three-inch gash between my wrist and knuckles.

The remainder of the route was far more perilous than what we'd negotiated so far: a few knife-edge ridges with 500-metre drops on either side, a handful of steep ice pitches, a tricky climb on ice and rock before reaching the peak at just over 4,000 metres, then a pant-filling descent on iced-over snow-slopes on the way to the next mountain hut. In the car the day before, we'd estimated the journey from hut to hut would take us ten hours. When we finally reached Rifugio Marco e Rosa, the mountain hut on the other, Italian side of the route, we'd been on the mountain for nineteen hours, not counting the hike in before our three hours of sleep in the Tschierva hut.

At Rifugio Marco e Rosa, we were greeted with a roar of applause by the teams of climbers who'd overtaken us on the route and witnessed our struggles to get Anders, and ourselves, off the mountain safely. Luigi had been complaining of chest pains since just before the summit, and while I was sleeping in the cramped dorm shared with sixteen others, David woke me to tell me he'd had a heart attack.

In the morning, the mountain-hut caretaker told us a helicopter would be on its way to airlift Luigi to the hospital in Sondrio shortly, but would only be able to take Luigi, not me or David. After finding another team to take Anders off the mountain, David and I rushed down the south side of the mountain over the Scerscen Glacier to the end of the road in Valmalenco, where he and Luigi had left Luigi's car on Friday night.

When we reached the car eight hours later and charged David's phone, we discovered the helicopter hadn't been able to land at the *rifugio* that morning owing to the high winds that had kicked up just as we were leaving. Luigi, however, was doing better. We drove directly to the hospital in Sondrio, hoping the chopper would have managed to land by the time we arrived, but when we called the *rifugio* again the caretaker told us they'd suspended the rescue until the next day. When we phoned the *rifugio* the next morning, they told us Luigi had decided to set off before sunrise to hike off the mountain under his own steam and they hadn't been able to dissuade him. He'd last been spotted assisting a duo of climbers struggling on the steep, ice-riddled couloir about half an hour south of the hut.

We drove up to the trailhead and parking area in Valmalenco and waited. After waiting for four hours, we spotted Luigi finally lumbering out of the larch-and-pine forest to the north, beyond which the trail up towards Piz Bernina wends over two high passes and across the Scerscen Glacier on its way to Rifugio Marco e Rosa, some 1,700 metres above.

I crossed the parking area to meet him with a hug and bottle of water.

His t-shirt was dripping with sweat. His face was pink and his lips cracked with sunburn.

'How are you?' I asked him. 'And what the hell happened up there?'

He took a long swig from the water bottle and steadied himself with an arm on my shoulder, then broke into a wide and jubilant smile.

'*L'alpinismo è sofferenza,*' he said.

'Anders was an idiot!' says Aiyla, who's never heard this story before.

'Maybe,' I say, 'but I understood him – his need to be up there, I mean. Even at seventy, even alone, even without the right gear. I understand him even more now. The absence devitalises you, wears you down. It's not like missing other things. It's not something you get used to; it just gets worse every day.'

'Is this what I have to look forward to?'

'What do you mean?'

'I mean waiting at home while you're away on three-day adventures trying to kill yourself?'

'Wait for me? You'll be coming too!'

Lockdown Day 7

The worst day.

Rain again.

While trying to read myself to sleep last night, I'd struck upon a plan: to walk to the supermarket to get around the no-walkabout-without-due-cause rule and get some fresh air and exercise. Three birds with one stone.

After breakfast, a mental image of Aiyla chiding me for my laxity sneaks into my morning meditation. I abandon the plan and resign myself to a day of work.

Others have been equally inventive. Dog-walking has exploded since the decree. Though I'm still avoiding social media, my WhatsApp groups have updated me on a dog-borrowing trend that's taken off nationwide. To keep things fair, or purely to lighten the mood, others have taken to walking their cats, gerbils and even goldfish.

My anticipated two-hour window of relief from work and boredom vanishes with the news that my football team's game against our Glasgow rivals has been cancelled. At last, my fellow Scots are seeing sense, but it doesn't appear infectious.

News arrives that China has donated thousands of masks and respirators to Italy in light of the national shortage. Instead of calming the uncalm, this segues into an uproar about the lack of assistance from our European neighbours. A story about the Slovenians building a wall on the Italian border doesn't help, despite countless Italians having proposed the exact-same measure to prevent Eastern European immigrants reaching Italy across the exact-same border just a few months ago. A British TV presenter accuses the Italians of wanting to take a national siesta, claiming the lockdown is just an excuse for absentee-ism. Dog walkers and others bold enough to post scenes from the outside world on social media are being attacked for their carelessness. Other Italian commentators see a racial divide in social-distancing efforts, posting photos of non-Caucasian citi-zens congregating in town squares, on park benches, on terraces outside closed bars, all while blithely ignoring the Caucasians out jogging, cycling, walking borrowed dogs and goldfish. The deaths caused by this virus will be mourned, but I do not know what will be done with the hatred.

I turn off my phone and lean back in my chair to gaze at the night. There's refuge even in the smallest and most distant trifles of nature – the stars, the stir of clouds, the blossoming harbingers of spring now peeping their heads above ground, as if to check where all the humans have gone.

Before bed I check the Worldometer stats again: Italy has 3,590 new cases and 368 new deaths.

Italy's death count is closing on China's in a race we don't want to win.

Lockdown Day 8

Monday. One week down, two and a half to go.

Over my morning coffee I allow myself my first daydream of what I'll do when this is all over. I'll take to the mountains and gorge myself on everything they offer: freedom, fresh air, beauty in abundance, a *sanctum sanctorum* far from the daily assault of information upon information, an unblemished canvas upon which I may stomp unhindered and uninterrupted for as long as my legs might carry me. Once that's taken care of, I'll fly to Istanbul and spend a week with Aiyla, then home to visit my parents, then New York to see my sister. I'll hug everyone I meet. I'll never again take for granted the simple act of going somewhere and the freedom to roam as I please. I'll ...

I should stop.

From my window I can see a total of eight peaks each over 2,300 metres high. I've climbed all eight of them, in both winter and summer. My favourite is Punta di Santo Stefano, a cupola-like point in the Alpi Orobie that stands at 2,697 metres. The peak directly in front of my bedroom window is the 2,374-metre Pizzo Meriggio. In my early days here, I used to park my car at 1,000 metres and jog up to the top for training, using snowshoes in winter. I must have climbed it at least thirty times. In my first few days of confinement, the mountains in view seemed to taunt me, but the urge to be up there among them has faded for now. I seem to be precisely where I should be.

My biggest fear is that when this is all over, it won't really be over, will it? When the authorities declare an end to the lockdown, who will return to their freedom as before? Who'll go hugging friends, shaking hands with strangers, kissing cheeks? Who'll travel, visit museums, go to concerts, go climbing? Who'll let their guard down in supermarkets, bars or cafés? Who'll do anything while there's even just one known case of this thing anywhere in the world at all?

Matteo calls. He's just returned from a week of work in Austria and was put through rigorous testing at the border upon re-entry. He tells me he's hunted through all the official rules and believes there's no blanket prohibition on walking for personal health. He thought of me when reading it, he says, and adds that he's seen people in his village heading up the mountain paths in the daytime, most of them dogless.

I've no sooner hung up than I abandon the idea of finishing off my work for the day and set off up the slopes of the mountain.

My initial nerves are quelled by sightings of three others, among them a jogger, and by the discovery that maintaining a distance of as much as five or ten metres is easily done on such a broad expanse of terrain. At one point an ex-student of mine jogs past on the trail. He sees me as he approaches, but he doesn't greet me and his eyes slide guiltily to the side as he passes.

I walk for three hours but don't feel the usual release. The pleasure of physical movement is tempered by my inability to shift thoughts of what the next few days and weeks, possibly months, will hold. The tension that has built up in increments over the last week seems to be lignifying my bones and muscles.

When I arrive home, the pot of soup I'd prepared earlier fails to stir my appetite. I head to bed early, willing the passing of another day towards the quarantine's end, like a kid counting the days to Christmas.

Lockdown Day 10

A cruelly beautiful day.

I miss my family and friends. It's starting to seem like I'll be missing them for quite some time.

I've travelled a lot and lived all over: Arizona, New Mexico, California, New York, Portugal, India, Nepal, Sicily, Trieste and, of course, Scotland. Though this peripatetic lifestyle has been the source of much joy, the lasting sentiment of my years on the road has been the heartbreak of leaving behind people whom I love and care about. It's the caveat that #wanderlust doesn't tell you about. I worry for them all, particularly those in the US and the UK, where the response has been like that of a drunkard waking to a fire in his house, saying, 'I'll deal with it later', and going back to sleep while his neighbours batter at his door.

From my window, I see a jogger on the winding street below the house. Ten seconds later: another. Before the rational part of my brain can veto me, I've dressed in running gear and am jogging slowly up the street towards the vineyards.

Before flying to visit Aiyla in Istanbul, I fractured my knee in a fall while climbing. The doctor told me there was slight ligament damage and I could expect to be sidelined from any serious activity for three months, at least. Above all else, he said, avoid jogging. When I went skiing with Lucia and the others before the lockdown, the pain was intense at times and I had to carry my skis on my back in one particularly steep gulley that would have required me to make numerous turns in the deep snow. Since then, I've been getting my daily exercise fix on the rowing machine and cross trainer in my apartment, both of which are a poor substitute for the real thing.

I am closing on the joggers as they approach the vineyards. There's a tall *palazzo* on the roadside on the way up, from where a woman calls from her window after the pair ahead of me: '*State a casa!*' (Stay at home!) They don't hear her, and luckily she's gone by the time I arrive.

As I pass the last of the houses and enter the vineyards, my fear subsides – if I see anyone out here, I'd have as much right to object as they would. The release is almost overpowering. The movement of my body is the purest joy. Countless little stimuli flicker as I pass beneath the trees and skirt through the narrow, rocky, labyrinthine trails between the sloping rows of vines, extending my gaze to the peaks of the Orobie and the tiny villages dotted along their flanks. In the gain-and-loss account of the past few weeks, perhaps I can add 'wonder' as the first positive.

On the third tier of vineyard I pass one of the two joggers I saw earlier. We flash massive grins at one another. I want to high-five her. Hug her, maybe. Tell her my life story. Instead, I continue, making plans for where to disburse all the unexpressed affection when this is all over.

An hour after I've returned home, my knee begins to throb. But even if I can't walk for the next week, it will have been worth it. My mood is better than it has been in days.

In the evening I avoid social media and instead read the news. The *Corriere della Sera* is reporting that, of nearly 200,000 Italians stopped and checked by the police, almost 10,000 have been fined for incorrect documentation or failure to observe the official decree. Meanwhile, a friend sends a picture to a WhatsApp group showing her in a jogging outfit on the streets of Trieste. She's lambasted by all, bar me.

I'm relieved to discover that the Brits and Americans are finally onboard with the appropriate containment and lockdown measures. I might see my family again after all.

Lockdown Day 11

The news reports 475 dead in a single day. *Four-seven-five*. That's roughly the population of my parents' village in

Scotland. The weight of this information seems to collect in my bones and I carry it around with me throughout the morning. Making coffee and opening my laptop seem barely within my powers.

Last night, the mayor of Milan and the minister for sport both threatened a blanket ban on leaving home for any reason without a *permesso*. Walkers and joggers were singled out for condemnation. I message Nicolò, the ex-student who'd ignored me as he jogged past in the vineyards yesterday, to find out what he knows about the rules put in place by the latest decree. In theory, he tells me, the ban hasn't been extended yet, but adds that the decree states people should only be walking and jogging if they have 'compelling' health reasons. He suffers from anxiety, he suddenly tells me, and has official permission from the doctor, but is now scared that he'll be attacked by vigilantes because of the growing antipathy towards anyone who is out, whether they have a bona fide *permesso* or not.

I choose to stay home rather than take my nightly walk in the vineyards. Though I'd like to tell myself my choice is motivated by a feeling of responsibility, I can't deny that it is inspired at least partially by a fear of repercussions. As 'compelling' as my reasons may be, one of the saddest realities of getting by with mental health issues in our times is the necessity of accepting that understanding, empathy and even basic recognition of the illnesses as valid health conditions are the exception, not the norm. Even if the state were to give us the green light for exercise, there would likely remain elements in the population at large unconvinced that we merit exemption.

So instead I wander idly around the garden until I get near the wall on the far side of the house. It's a 50-foot-long,

8-foot-tall affair made of lumps of flaky schist and gneiss along with square-foot blocks of serpentine and granite from the quarries in Valmalenco. I've never paid the wall much attention when cutting the grass or at my kitchen window. From there, it's partially hidden by the last few vines and appears to be a wall like any other in the *cittavecchia*, the old town – antiquated, slightly dilapidated and with a sort of makeshift ruggedness that somehow makes it all the more aesthetically endearing. But after I climb the thirty or so steps from the front of the house to inspect it more closely, I see there's more to it. The multicoloured stones are set in concrete, almost haphazardly, and each one features a rounded or serrated edge that protrudes far enough to take at least a few fingertips or a toe. I rub my hands over their alternately coarse (granite, gneiss) and slick (serpentine, schist) surfaces, giving a tug here and there to test their stability. Some come out without any resistance, but the majority seem well embedded and sturdy enough to bear weight – maybe as much as my 80-something kilogrammes.

I run inside and fetch my climbing shoes, then end up spending two hours traversing back and forth along the wall, finding more pleasure than I ever thought possible from something so banal. It's a far cry from the 2,000-foot walls of Val di Mello, Valmasino and Valmalenco that I'd hoped to be climbing this month, but by the end of the first traverse I think I might have found the source of my salvation for as long as the others remain off-limits.

When I finish, I stay in the garden, sitting on the short patch of untended lawn watching the sun set behind the Orobie and imbibing the miasma of scents, the signifiers of a spring that knows nothing of the catastrophe unfolding within its embrace.

The cherry blossoms are already falling.

Italy has passed the Chinese death toll already.

Lockdown Day 12

Friday.

At 3 p.m. I knock off work and go to sit in the garden. I choose a tree stump that faces out over the *cittavecchia*, a slim vein of stone-built and slate-roofed terraced buildings to either side of Via Scarpatetti, the neighbourhood's cobbled central thoroughfare and centre of activity. Now, no one passes there, and the only vehicles are police cars checking for anyone in breach of *quarantena*. My neighbour's goats provide the only punctuation to the steady wail of sirens and the drone of the helicopter doing its rounds up and down the valley. Below, I see another neighbour, Fausto, tending to his vegetable plot in a small enclosure below the vineyards. His mother, Elvira, died last year. While I was still a teacher, she would appear at her door in her pinafore every morning at 8.56, with flour- or polenta-specked hands, to give me *baci* on my way to my 9 a.m. class. Since the first time she didn't appear, Fausto has spent every day in the plot, tending to his tomatoes and lettuces and carrots with his coterie of chickens.

I have little doubt that the Valtellina valley is the most heavenly spot on Earth. When I first arrived, my new boss picked me up from Bergamo Airport and drove me to a hotel in Sondrio. We passed various famous tourist hotspots on the way – Lake Como, Varenna, Lecco – then rounded the curve past the town of Morbegno into the wide berth of Valtellina proper, where a colonnade of tall peaks on either side framed the glistening outline of Monte Adamello – the Adamello

Massif – in the distance. I knew I was home. After almost twenty years of wandering the planet in search of some suitable terminus, funding the venture as an itinerant teacher of English, arriving here was as much a relief as it was joy. Everything I saw appeared to be precisely where it should be, almost as if it matched a blueprint in my subconscious. That intuition grew with time. I could never have dreamed of a more suitable place for myself. I had mountains galore. I had enough climbing crags to visit one each day of the year and still have a few left over. Soon, I had climbing partners whose passion and energy were inexhaustible. I had the peace and quiet and absence of harsh stimuli needed to mitigate and control my Bipolar and its various side effects. I had friends whose warmth and humanity humbled me. On my travels I always felt like I was missing out on something, but here I'm *in* that something.

The greatest of anything is that which you simply can't explain or rationalise. Anything that can be said can equally be unsaid; anything explained can be explained away; anything enumerated just as easily subtracted. If I am depressed because of circumstance – illness, unemployment, bereavement – then that depression might be cured more easily; if I am depressed with no reason, then I'm in trouble. Great love is no different. If I say 'I love her because . . .', the 'because' can be negated, demoted, or might wane. If I have no notion of why I love her, however, then it's just there. That's how I feel about Valtellina. Although it possesses all of the elements I love – mountains, culture, good people, pizza, strong coffee, snow, ice and rock – these are conveniences. Practicalities. Credentials. Over and above, there is an unconditional attachment and affection that is far more binding.

The biggest threat to my stay in Valtellina came in the form of a girl. She was the kind of girl for whom most men would climb mountains. The only trouble was, she didn't climb mountains. Nor did she have much appreciation for just looking at them or being in their presence. Six months into our relationship, I came home from work one day and found on my kitchen table a list of job openings in the area in Portugal to which she wished to relocate. With it came an ultimatum: leave Valtellina or leave her. She is now a happily married resident of Sines, Alentejo.

Giuseppina appears on her balcony but doesn't see me. I choose not to disturb her, even though I know this time will be weighing heavily on her more than most and she wants for company. Domenico, her husband, was the type of man who could leave you in stitches with just a glance, and as kind as humans are made. Though well into his tenth decade, he used to come downstairs to check on me and ask if he could help with anything.

I remember standing with him on that same balcony a few months before his death from heart failure. We were looking out over the town, discussing how it had changed in the past fifty years, when we heard voices from the street.

'Ah, yes,' he said, nodding towards a trio of elderly men gathered just beyond the front gate. 'Do you see? They know I'm for it. These chancers are already lining up to be Giuseppina's toy boy once I'm gone, the rascals! I'll come back and haunt the lot of them, I tell you.'

I message an ex-colleague, Holly, who lives around 150 metres from my apartment. She teaches in a school in Morbegno, around 15 miles west of Sondrio, and I haven't heard from her since the outbreak began. She replies minutes later, telling me she has bronchitis. She hasn't been to the hospital for testing because she knows there are no tests to be had.

Lockdown Day 13

Saturday again.

There is, every day, a gorgeous two-second window upon awakening when the world is as it was.

Then the silence . . .

Then the ambulance sirens.

Then the hum of the air-ambulance choppers.

The *Corriere della Sera* newspaper reports 3,654 infected nurses nationwide. Seventeen doctors have died. Holly's illness reveals how the official statistics on infected cases are likely understated. If there was merely one Holly for every *comune* (municipality) in the region, then the tally of the infected would swell by another 1,500 in Lombardy alone. The likelihood is that each *comune* harbours at least a dozen or more Hollys who have mild symptoms or are asymptomatic. There are 7,982 *comuni* in Italy.

In response to the high death toll posted in the last few days, the government has now extended the ban on *spostamenti* ('movements'). Walking and jogging are now out. Unequivocally. In keeping with the Italian fetish for paperwork, the government has released a third version of the self-certification document required for anyone leaving their home for any purpose.

My social media is flooded with images of students on spring break in Miami and Australia, and of Brits enjoying their last weekend in pubs before lockdown. My feelings take a straight 50:50 split, one part considering their actions tantamount to criminal negligence, the other sympathising with their ignorance and inability to comprehend the magnitude of the crisis and the possible consequences of everything any of us do now or in the coming months.

If ignorance is a defence, how many of us could claim shelter? Maybe none; maybe all. Misinformation has played a role in virtually every significant event in the past decade, and this pandemic is no exception. The scale and severity of the situation may also be too much for our brains to fathom. We've never seen anything like it. As historical eras go, the twenty-first century has not been good preparation for crisis. We've become habituated to ease, expectant of progress, weaned on such slogans as #liveyourbestlife. The average twenty-first-century citizen in developed countries is so accustomed to leisure and getting things their way that a pandemic is an unimaginable rupture.

Meanwhile, the local news is dominated by the story of three hikers who broke quarantine to walk a path above the village of Spriana in Valmalenco, around five miles away. One of them fell and broke an ankle and had to be airlifted to the hospital. The backlash from their fellow citizens began before the chopper had even touched down on the helipad on the hospital roof.

People are beginning to ask why Italy has been so hard-hit. The slight delay in imposing the lockdown, and the imbecility of all those probable vectors who fled to the south in the final hours before the quarantine became official, is partially responsible, as is the high percentage of Italians over the age of sixty-five. But the figures posted by other European nations – Germany, Belgium and Norway, in particular – convince me that the most compelling argument lies in the influence of national habits and conventions.

Italians are gregarious people. They are far more touchy-feely than northern Europeans and even other southern Europeans. They hug more, kiss more, pet more. One abiding memory from my first years here, whether in Palermo, Trieste or here in Sondrio, was the culture shock of discovering the national absence of spatial awareness. On trains I'd find it hard to determine where my leg ended and my neighbour's began. In supermarkets I became used to the front of the next shopper-in-line's trolley resting under my buttocks. In narrow streets, I learned to account for those blocking the way letting me get to within a few inches, pausing to examine me, and greeting me before letting me pass. I soon came to see these invasions of my space as an extension of the Italians' genuine warmth and sociability. None of these habits, however, help social distancing and the containment of a virus that's passed person-to-person. In that critical period when the virus first appeared in Italy, moreover, no moratorium was declared on physical closeness until long after the virus had flown the few isolated hotspots in the north and spread south.

Aiyla video-calls while I'm having breakfast. The numbers of cases and deaths in Turkey are now accelerating at a similar rate to those of Italy in the early days. She and her family have decided to continue self-isolating, despite the government still maintaining a fairly relaxed official containment policy.

'Tell me how you're doing,' she says. Though Aiyla is a psychologist, she rarely bothers to assess my mental state, but on the odd occasion that she does, her voice is more pointed, different, while trying not to be. Like now.

'I'm fine,' I say, trying to sound as fine as possible.

'No, you're not. You're not sleeping. You've lost weight. Your face is . . . what's the word?'

She makes a face like a fish.

'Drawn?'

'Yes, drawn.'

'Maybe.'

'So?'

I feel like I'm on the start of a climb that's above my pay grade. I can turn back and avoid the discomfort, or soldier on and maybe feel a sense of achievement afterwards.

'It's hard,' I say, setting off on impulse before I've thought through the route ahead.

'What is, exactly?'

'The deaths. The people dying. There's so many.'

'Yes.'

'There will be a lot more, too. I know that.'

'Does it make you feel afraid?'

'No. Not afraid. Just sad. Helpless, maybe. Useless. I tried to volunteer for the Red Cross today, but they've suspended the training courses. I want to help somehow.'

'Kieran, you can't. You have to think about Giuseppina too. She's never more than a few metres away from you. And she's high-risk.'

'Yeah, I know.'

'Okay, so let's think. What more could you do to help the situation?'

'Nothing, I guess. That's the point.'

'Yes. Are you feeling lonely or isolated?'

'A bit, maybe. But I'm turning my phone off each day and rejecting calls; I don't really want to speak to anyone, but I'm lonely, too. It's hard to explain. When I see someone in the street or in the supermarket, I become almost tearful. I have this urge to hug them, to speak to them, even if they're 200 yards away and might be someone who voted for Lega.'

'Lega?'

'The nationalist separatist party. The ones who want to build a wall north of Bologna. They're Italy's version of Trump's Republicans, or of Turkey's Erdogan fans.'

She doesn't laugh.

'Why do you turn your phone off?'

'To block it out, maybe. So I can immerse myself in work and find more of the moments when I forget this is happening.'

'Are you able to work, to write your articles?'

'Not like before. It takes me twice as long, even though I have nothing else to do.'

'What would make you feel better?'

'You mean, besides the virus suddenly dying off and life returning to how it was?'

'Yep.'

'I don't know. A hug, maybe. Less anger. A little bit of light at the end of the tunnel.'

'Well, we can't do anything about the hug. But we can help with the anger – just switch off from it. Use your phone only to work for you, to give you an outlet and let you check on the people you care about – nothing else. If you had kept it off from day one and only called me and your family, you would've known nothing about all that anger. How do you think you'd be feeling now if that was the case?'

'Better,' I say, cringing ever so slightly with the awareness that I'm a journalist advocating ignorance.

'What do you do when you wake during the night? How do you feel?'

'Anxious. I check my phone to read the news.'

'Why? What are you looking for?'

'Some good news. Anything.'

'You can't depend on that now, not for your happiness and calm. You have to find other ways.'

'Yup, I know.'

'Are you worried? About how this will affect you, I mean.'

'Nah, not yet.'

'You know, you've never really told me what it's like. When it's really bad, I mean.'

'I have.'

'"Shite" covers a lot of things, granted, but it doesn't really paint much of a picture.'

'No, not really.'

'So?'

'It's hard to explain.'

Each time it feels like setting up camp in a cul-de-sac. Even if there were anything worth describing, the dullness of it robs you not only of the energy and will to do so but also the very words with which you'd do the describing.

'Try. I don't want to use a pandemic as an excuse to dive into your psyche or anything, but it would be good for me to know, don't you think?'

'Aiyla ...'

'Come on! Every time you shut me down on this you say, "It's a long story" or, "It's hardly dating chat." Well, now we've got a lot of time on our hands, we're well past the dating stage, and it might just help me to help you.'

'It's not hard to talk about because it's painful to dredge up – that too, of course – but more because the words are never there. And it's always too easy to downplay it. Make light of it. I don't know why. Maybe shame. Maybe because each time you hope you've moved on and it'll never happen again. Maybe because by talking about it seriously you admit it's real and let it poison even normal times.'

'If the words aren't there now because you're in a different place, how about you read me the ones you used when you *were* there?'

'You mean my diaries?'

Since I was a teenager, writing a daily diary has been one of the ways I've managed to offload and defuse whatever's been going on in my head. I have dozens of the things stashed in a box in my room.

'If you'd feel comfortable doing that, that is.'

I go and fetch my diaries.

'Okay.'

Edinburgh, June 2004

A neon light beckons from the town below. Voices rise through the valleys of rooftops, summons to something only known in memory. Forgetting myself, I'm drawn by some dormant instinct down from the hill and into their midst. I'm soon in the city streets, joining the quiet procession of dinner-time passers-by, clocked-off workers hurrying home on the sigh of a day's end.

My feet take me into the town centre. I pass couples arm-in-arm, dog walkers, coffee-shop windows framing polite bourgeois Scenes of Earth.

I belonged here once, before 'It All'. My visits now are like to a childhood home – the family inside no longer my own, despite my expectation, and each memory a petite madeleine *coated in salt, barbed with the bitterness of that cardinal, constitutive injustice around which life has revolved.*

Standing in front of those windows, I am reminded of why I had gone to the hill. Not for solitude so much as to forget.

Down here I am both haunter and haunted, interloper and exile. With a heavy heart, I retrace my steps, counting the changes wrought, the Thens and Nows. The longing. The non-negotiable acceptance of unbidden experience. The forsaken simplicity. The otherness.

And the window. Always the window . . .

New Mexico, February 2008

If walls could talk: 'He lay on the floor all day again.'

Manali, India, September 2011

Another room. I've had at least a dozen of them now. Places where I've gone to die awhile while the world goes on without me.

I've been here a week. Seems no point in saying how long. Time's irrelevant when there's no future.

There is no future.

Even if there were, what will remain of the world when this one's over? How many friends will be left this time?

I'm not strong enough for this any more – life. Lives, even. I feel like I've lived a hundred of them and yet I've got nowhere, lost everything, gained nothing but battle wounds that only remind me of defeat after defeat after . . .

I am a geographical anomaly, ravaged now by storms, now by floods, now by droughts and wildfire. In the interims, every attempt at amends is futile.

What's the point in getting back up and starting over if you're biologically programmed to oversee and orchestrate your own downfall every time?

Mosstowie, Scotland, February 2013

I have three rocks: the figurative, human kind; the literal, climbable kind; the consumable, pharmaceutical kind that comes in a blister pack. I realise now that I need all three – take any one of them away and I'll crumble.

Lundin Links, Scotland, December 2010

When the lights go out there isn't darkness. Darkness would be a blessing, the slightest hazing of the horror of humanness the greatest kindness imaginable.

A week ago I'd owned the world. There was a near-mystical unity with everything I encountered. Now everything is atomised. Everything is a stranger to everything else. The cruelty of the division is how the accounting's done. When up, down is impossible but also inevitable. When down, happiness is a dream of which I'm undeserving and that will never return.

I close the last of the diaries and put it away in the box.

'Thank you,' says Aiyla, who's remained silent all the time I've been reading.

'It's a start . . .'

'A start?'

'Yeah, well, I obviously didn't get to . . . you know, the bit we never talk about.'

'You mean . . . suicide.'

'Yeah, of course. They say around one in seventy people have Bipolar at some point in their life and a third of them are likely to try suicide. And the suicide rate's twenty times higher for Bipolars than for Normals. So . . .'

'You can go on. I'm happy to know as much as you're willing to tell.'

'Well, people are always surprised. But for us Bipolars, their surprise is surprising. Because it's the most logical thing ever, isn't it? I often think about the difference between symptoms of illness and consequences of illness. The symptoms of heart disease are clogged and narrowing arteries. At a certain point, the disease to the heart reaches a "critical mass" and the heart packs in. The symptoms of Bipolar or any other mental illness are suffering. At a certain point, when the suffering's reached a critical mass, the sufferer packs in too. That just makes sense, right? The only people who think there's any volition involved, or that one's less automatic than the other, are those who've never been there. Because when you're there, it's just *there*. You think there's no way back or forward, only in or out. Then when you get past it, you look back and you don't feel good that it's gone; you just think about whether next time the suffering will take you one step further. A final step, I mean.'

'Now I'm worried.'

'Don't be. That's part of why it's hard to talk about – people worrying when they have no reason to. And you have no reason to, I promise. I have my rocks, after all. I can speak to you, Ma, Pa and Cath the same as always. I've got meds. And if I can get out on Giuseppina's wall every day, I'll have a passable version of all three. They'll let me keep it together for a few weeks, I'm sure. I'm just riding out the storm.'

I return to the garden and find Giuseppina there with her daughter, Cristina. Giuseppina's sitting on the swing-chair beneath my living room window and Cristina's on a camping chair on the lawn. Both are dressed in winter jackets though the temperature must be north of 20 degrees, the sun high above the clouds crowded around the head of Pizzo Meriggio. They ask me to join them. I fetch my mask from inside and take a seat on the wall enclosing the small rectangle of grass between the house and the vineyard, making sure I'm near enough that Giuseppina can hear me and far enough away that I needn't fear passing on the virus should I have become infected on my trip to the supermarket.

Cristina tells me of her cousin near Bergamo, whose husband was taken into hospital after testing positive for the virus. Due to the lack of beds and even corridor space, he wasn't taken into the nearest hospital and the cousin now no longer knows where he is or even whether he's dead or alive.

'It's happening everywhere!' she says. 'This, I tell you, is quintessentially Italian. We have a million departments responsible for everything under the sun but every one of them tells you it's not their responsibility and passes the buck to the next. The poor woman's been on the phone all day to every hospital and crematorium within 50 kilometres!'

While Cristina is speaking, Giuseppina sits on the swing-chair in her faded sunhat, looking out over the town and valley. She has her hearing aid on, but I know she gave up trying to follow the conversation some time ago. I wonder how it must be for her, ninety years into a life lived entirely within 100 metres of where she's sitting, to now be faced with this.

The bell tower tolls three.

Monica, the youngest of Giuseppina's three daughters, appears with Enzo, her husband, and soon we have formed a wide circle across which we yell our news and the stories we've heard in the past few days. The talk is dominated by our mutual confoundment. From the innocence of just three weeks ago to ... *this*. Two hours pass. When the church bell tolls five I realise we've all sat in silence for the past ten minutes. Silence is not the Italian way. There is always something to be said, some positive spin. There are footnotes upon footnotes, asides upon asides. Now, we've exhausted every avenue. But there is a solidarity. We are joined by a common enemy, a common cause, a common care for each other's well-being and helplessness to do anything more than sit and be together. I look around at each of their faces and realise something that has never come to me in the six years I've been here: this is also my family.

Lockdown Day 14

I didn't sleep. Waking around midnight, I shuffled around the apartment, going between my bookshelves looking for something to read, checking the news, tidying already tidied clothes and putting them in separate bundles. There's no more housework left to do.

I take a seat to the window and draw up a list of reasons to remain positive:

1. I am still alive.
2. My family and friends are still alive.
3. I am healthy and so are my family and friends.
4. Video chat allows me to speak with my family and friends and to know they are alive and well in a time that would otherwise be unbearably bleak.

Kieran Cunningham

5. I can work through the pandemic, writing articles for hiking, climbing and camping websites that haven't suspended activity, and avoid the uncertain future faced by so many others.
6. Netflix.
7. The mountains will still be there when this is all over.
8. This has probably been good for my dodgy knee, allowing it to recover in a way I wouldn't have let it had there been no lockdown.
9. I have seven unread books on my shelves.
10. I found a pack of peanut-butter cookies at the back of my biscuit cupboard.
11. I quit smoking one year and seven months ago.
12. I live in a place where the healthcare system is outstanding and free.
13. I've caught up with friends I haven't spoken to in years and might otherwise never have spoken to again.
14. The genuine smiles of those I've passed on my rare trips to the supermarket.
15. I have a garden and am not confined to an apartment in a city, where I would surely fare far worse.
16. The cherry blossoms and wisteria are flowering in the garden.
17. The wall of Giuseppina's house, which has in the last few days become my climbing gym and greatest source of consolation and means of coping.
18. Giuseppina, whose strength and imperturbable stoicism are a great inspiration.
19. The adaptability of our species: while I have no wish for this to become normal, I can feel I'm making the

52

situation more liveable with each day that passes and see others doing likewise.

20. Perspective: the big things that normally dominate our lives are no longer there, so we have more attention, more bandwidth, to give to the little things. For every bit of news dissected and pored over in fine detail, every shudder of horror, every fear-inspired outburst on social media, there is a flower, an insect, a gorgeous chink of light through an open curtain that we might not have seen and marvelled at otherwise.

21. I'm thirty-eight years old. Had this happened fifteen or even ten years ago, when I wasn't so attuned to the onset of my episodes, this situation would've been a lot scarier by far. I've had to adopt a kind of siege mentality and become extra-vigilant, upping my meditation times and watching myself for any of the usual signs – increased heart rate, compulsiveness, jumpiness, distractibility, trembling hands, excitability, questionable purchases on Amazon and eBay – that a manic episode might be in the offing, but there's a kind of comfort in knowing that I'm now better equipped to do that than ever before.

22. I have a choice: accept, act or suffer. I cannot act. Suffering is suboptimal. Acceptance is the only way.

In the morning I hear from Holly. She's no better. A doctor visited her yesterday and told her she is developing either pneumonia or the virus, but couldn't say which. Swab tests are being limited to only critically ill patients, so he's organised a blood test to check her count of white cells: high means pneumonia, low means the virus.

Aiyla calls next, from her balcony, where she's gone to get some peace from her family. The number of prayer calls from her local mosque has increased tenfold in the past week. Most of the calls, she says, are funerary. Though the Turkish government has belatedly released some statistics on infections and deaths, she suspects these figures are vastly understated.

It's Mother's Day in the UK. I call my mum. She and Pa are now self-isolating, though the rest of Britain appears to be at the seaside.

'I've taken up yoga,' Ma tells me. 'Me and your dad were doing it together this morning. It'll be good for his hip, I think, and I'm enjoying it. With all the baking I've been doing, I need to be doing some exercise so you won't have to roll me out of the house when this is all over.'

'That's great, Ma.'

'Well, we're all doing what we can, aren't we? I speak to your aunty Brenda every day, and your uncles, and Moira next door speaks to me over the wall. Your sister had a three-way with Chris and Ryan yesterday.'

'She—?'

'You know, when the three of you chat by video together on the What's Up. We could all do that – you in Italy, your sister in New York, and me and your dad here.'

'Ah, yes. But if you speak to anyone else about it please tell them she's video-chatting, okay?'

'What? Why?'

'Never mind. What about walking? Can't you take Rufus along the beach? If you go at low tide you can give anyone down there a wide berth.'

'I'm too worried. Everyone else seems to be going about

their business as usual, but I wouldn't be able to relax. So I'm just going to stay home and try not to kill your father.'

'How is he?'

'Envious of your wall. Regretting ignoring your recommendation of making that artificial climbing wall on the side of the house with those coloured thingies, like in the gym in Ratho.'

'Put him on.'

She puts him on.

He tries to sound upbeat but the effort is all too apparent. The cause of his ennui is easy to guess.

'You're still getting deliveries, right?' I ask him. 'Just order a bunch of holds online and put them around the shed. Traverse around that a few times a day and you'll be okay.'

'You think your mother will let me?'

'Nah, absolutely not. Get out there and drill the holes while she's watching *Emmerdale*, then fit the bolts during *EastEnders*.'

'I'll think about it. I've barely retired; it'd be a pity to get myself killed now. Anyway, how are you holding up?'

'I'm getting through it. It's not so bad as it was at the start . . . I'm finding ways to make it more liveable.'

'Glad to hear it. I'm thinking about you. You know that, right?'

'I do. Don't worry about me. Just look after yourself and Ma.'

I put in a few hours' work before my brain declares itself spent. Now restricted to exercising on my own property, I jog up and down the lanes of Giuseppina's vineyard in my lunchbreak until my knee is too painful to continue. Before dinner, I spend an hour climbing the wall of the house and another hour raking and bagging fallen leaves in the garden. It's starting to dawn on me how fortunate I am. The garden, the vineyard, the climbable wall, the rock star of a landlady looking out for me every day, the views of the mountains at every window. Take away any of them and my life in lockdown would be a whole lot less tolerable.

Lockdown Day 15

I may be losing it.

The glue that's been holding me together has been the assumption that this will all be over soon. I mean, 3 April – the scheduled end of *quarantena* – is only a few weeks away and China has already been posting 'no new case' days regularly, even in Wuhan, the pandemic's source. April 3rd seemed optimistic and unrealistic from the outset, but I'd been hoping that by early May, or June at worst, normality would have been restored at least in part. That glue's undoing has been the realisation that the quarantine will continue far beyond even that; that nobody will be out of this until we're *all* out of it – something more likely to take a year than a month.

It's 3 a.m. I've been awake for an hour or so, sitting in the kitchen, listening to the wind. The church bells chime as always. Two strikes, two and a ding, three strikes, three and a ding ... The wind is blowing from the east, purring in the boughs of magnolia blossom.

When I look down at my hand, I notice it's shaking. I trudge to the bathroom for my meds, pop one and count the rest. Sixteen left. The postal service has been paused so I decide to ration them to one every two days. Maybe the post will resume soon and Ma can send a new supply then.

Last spring I had an episode that culminated with a night

revelling in the interplay of the stars and the leaves of the Japanese maple in the garden, where I collapsed from exhaustion a short time later. I went to see a specialist in Edinburgh while home visiting my parents in the summer and we agreed that I should resume using lithium.

The episode was my first in over a year and had scared the shit out of me; not the end result – the collapse, the night in hospital, and the week I'd spent in bed dependent on friends and, eventually, my mother to feed me – but rather the weeks prior, in which I'd had no control over my increasingly reckless and unhinged behaviour. At the end of it all, I'd looked back at everything I'd done – crashed my car, painted poetry on the living room walls in huge, purple letters, solo-climbed three difficult mountain routes on three different nights, alone and in the dark – and was unable to consider myself the agent of any of it.

This is the scariest part: the inability to remain aware enough to stop myself doing things that, in normal times, would be unthinkable and entirely out of character; things that might, at best, result in serious injury or, at worst, put my parents on the receiving end of a phone call telling them their son's been in a car accident, gone missing, or is on his way down a mountain in a body bag. In the early days of my condition, when I was carless and living in areas whose topography boasted landmarks no more fearful than the sub-300-metre grassy lumps of Arthur's Seat and Largo Law, the feelings of invincibility I experience weren't such a problem. Here, having a veritable shit-ton of 3,000-metre-plus peaks, 500-metre monoliths and climbing crags by the dozen all within easy driving distance in my aged Fiat Panda, misadventure-avoidance is more of a concern.

The awareness only comes with hindsight, by which point I

can usually expect to find myself standing at yet another personal ground zero, having ruined or lost everything I'd had before the episode struck – friendships, relationships, jobs and most of my faith in the point or worth of starting over. It's like rebuilding a life between hurricanes and floods, each time knowing that every effort might be in vain. The episode last spring wasn't bad, relatively speaking, and didn't scare me as much as previous ones – I'd changed meds shortly beforehand and could easily put the mania down to teething problems or delayed readjustment – but it also reminded me that, regardless of how stable I'd been in Sondrio until then, changes in circumstance, whatever their nature, were still liable to put that stability in jeopardy.

'As long as you take these, and keep getting your climbing, walking and fresh air,' the doctor in Edinburgh had told me, 'I'm sure you'll be just fine.'

I returned to Italy with enough meds to see me through the next few months. After Christmas I'd gone to visit a doctor in Sondrio. I could have gone to her directly for help before this, but communicating the experience of episodes is tricky enough in your mother tongue, let alone your second. The doctor was happy to accept the specialist's prescription, but told me I'd have to redo the blood tests to be issued with the meds in Italy. She also warned me that neither the blood test nor the medication would be cheap. As a foreign resident, I'd have to make a con-tribution, one that – I discovered when she scribbled the sum on her notebook and spun it towards me – I was too poor to pay. My bank account was only just beginning to recover from the near-fatal hit it had taken as a result of that spring episode, during which I'd had to start selling off my climbing gear and living on tinned tuna just to get through the month. With my ticket already booked, I told her I'd come back and sort it all out as soon as I got back from visiting my girlfriend in Turkey, unaware that a pandemic was brewing and would have touched down in Italy by the time I returned.

At noon there's a knock on my door. I can't believe there's a knock on my door. I sit still and listen to make sure I'm not imagining things.

There's another knock on my door.

I put on my mask and turn the key, taking a step back as I swing the door open. It's Giuseppina, holding a plate of freshly sliced bresaola, a staple of our pre-coronavirus lunches upstairs. I've been eating pre-cooked chicken, tinned tuna and tins of chickpeas garnished with mayonnaise for the last two weeks, having stocked up on long-lasting fare only in order to minimise trips to the supermarket – and because the thought of enjoying anything, food included, somehow feels like a dereliction of empathy, given the global mood. I'm salivating before I have the chance to thank her.

'I thought you were looking thin, yesterday. You must eat, *ragazzo*!'

Her smile is a miracle. Her visit, however, worries me.

'Are you doing okay?' I ask her.

She shrugs and smiles.

'I do as I do. I have pains in my neck and my hips. But it will pass. Everything will pass.'

She blows me a kiss and waves goodbye. Halfway up the steps to her door she stops and calls back.

'If you need anything, let me know.'

It's 3 p.m. and I've had no reply from Holly to a message I sent this morning. I take a break from work and try calling.

No answer. I text a few other former colleagues from the school then go into the garden and wander between the trees and flowers while I wait for a reply.

One of my neighbour's goats spots me by the fence and trots over to greet me. I pluck a handful of the overgrown grass on our side of the fence and drop it over beside him. When he's finished, he taps his nose on the fence until I tear another few handfuls and drop them over too. While he's munching, I pull out my phone and google 'Can animals transmit coronavirus?' The first few results suggest no. I grab another handful of grass, feed it to him by hand, then lean over the fence and wrap my arms around him. He smells faintly of urine and wet hay, but I don't mind. It's the first hug I've given in two weeks. It feels, frankly, awesome, even with his rock-like horns pressing into my solar plexus and their pointed tips resting marginally below my throat. He doesn't resist, but soon gives a little nod to tell me he's ready for more grass.

A reply comes in from the secretary at Holly's school: her situation hasn't improved and a doctor has gone to her apartment to do blood tests.

Before I can digest this, a call comes in from my mother. My cousin, Eric, has the virus. I call his wife. Nervous by nature, she's uncharacteristically calm and resigned to the inevitability of catching the virus herself. They separated six months ago but as soon as he became unwell she returned to his side. If anything good comes out of this thing, it will be hundreds of newly crowned heroes like her, the counterweight to the attention-starved conspiracy theorists, racists, xenophobes and self-appointed spokespersons milking every opportunity to spew their anger.

That night, I call Aiyla. She's incensed by the news from the US, where the president has defied the counsel of all qualified advisers and announced that America will 'reopen' soon.

'It's just confirmation,' she says, 'that money is more valuable than human life. I don't know where to fit that in my world view.'

'Yep,' I say. 'Here they're handing out masks by the dozen to footballers and telling the nurses to reuse the same ones they've been using for weeks.'

'Everything we've known for so long is crystallising, isn't it? It's devastating.'

'Maybe it will be the start of the turnaround. I mean, maybe it will wake people up.'

She gets changed for bed while we speak.

'What?' she says, between slipping out of her jeans and sweater and into her pyjamas.

I realise I've been silent, staring, possibly drooling.

'Eh, nothing,' I say.

'I know,' she says, after throwing on a t-shirt, 'I feel it too.'

'Feel what?' I ask, fumbling my attempt to play dumb.

'Sex. The lack of it.'

'Yeah, well, there's not much we can do, is there?'

'Phone sex?'

'Hmmmm. Let's maybe bank that one for later. Now doesn't really seem like the time, what with my cousin being nearly dead and my neighbours dropping like flies and all.'

'Of course. I was joking. We'll just have to make up for it when this is all over.'

'That would require another kind of quarantine, maybe longer than this one.'

She laughs. 'Don't flatter yourself!'

Her laugh is like a firework every time, a small explosion that lights up everything within a 20-metre radius.

'Go sleep, Viking,' she says. '*Tatli ruyalar.*'

'*Tatli ruyalar*, Midget.'

'We'll get through this, won't we?'

'Of course we will.'

Lockdown Day 16

Tuesday.

My apartment has a new tenant. I caught sight of him/her this morning – a tiny mobile smudge of brown on the white tiles below the kitchen sink, scuttling around the skirting before diving into a tiny gap under a cupboard. A field mouse. Each morning for the past week I've found his droppings in various corners around the apartment. I ping a few crumbs of cereal into the gap in the skirting, glad to have any kind of company that can't be considered a potential vector.

Amazing what can happen in twenty-four hours on Earth. In addition to Trump's announcement of his new, kamikaze-style approach to pandemic containment, the UK has finally imposed a lockdown, just hours after countless photos and reports emerged of thousands of people flocking to popular spots in the Highlands and along the coast and defying the prohibition on social gatherings, inspired by the unseasonably warm March weather. In the meantime, Spain has posted a record-high death toll of 462 and the press is reporting on old people in care homes being abandoned or found dead in their beds. In Colombia, rebel fighters and paramilitary groups have used the lockdown to start killing off the nation's activists. Hungary is on the verge of giving its far-right leader the right to rule by decree. Drones and cell phones are being used to track whether citizens of various nations, Italy included, are complying with quarantine. Cuba, China and Russia have sent doctors to help with the crisis in Italy, while Germany has admitted six critically ill Italian patients to stem the tidal wave flooding into Italian hospitals.

I put in an hour of gardening and then take my morning coffee onto the terrace. The high winds of yesterday have scattered more magnolia petals across the lawn, leaving the tree all but bare. The sky is purest milk, a huddle of clotted clouds hung low over the valley. Giuseppina's door clicks open. I look up to see if she's there and soon her head appears over the staircase.

'Wait,' she says.

I wait. A few minutes later she returns with a coffee of her own and pulls a chair onto the landing at the top of the stairs.

'Like that we can have a bit of company. I can't hear you, but we can just sit.'

We just sit. The sun slowly burns through the clouds. Birds flit from tree to tree around us, cacophonous in their morning song.

'I'm afraid I can't offer you anything because I might give you the virus,' she calls down, attempting to use the English pronunciation of the word, which for some reason has become de rigueur in all Italian news outlets.

'Aren't you working today?' she adds.

'Later,' I yell back, scaring the shit out of a lizard who's scuttled to within a few feet of my chair to take the morning sun.

'It is good that you work. It gives you a meaning. My father always told me there's nobility in working. But don't overdo it.'

She returns her gaze to the dispersing clouds.

She and Domenico built this house in 1957. The plot of land had been owned by her family for more than three centuries. Until then, she'd lived in one of the houses below the vineyard on Via Scarpatetti – a three-storey, stone-built *palazzo* with iron lattice over the street-level windows, external staircases and precarious-looking balconies made with huge, contorted wood beams, and a faded fresco along the facade. The next five houses on either side had been occupied by her grandparents, uncles, aunts and cousins. She told me her great-grandfather had built the Scarpatetti house with a large cellar specially for the animals; when she was a young girl, the family would spend winter nights in there with the sheep and goats, for warmth. She'd met Domenico while she was training as a dressmaker. He was a bank clerk in the original Banca Popolare building in Piazza Garibaldi, the town square. Ten years her senior, he was eligible for the draft when Italy entered the Second World War. Unwilling to fight for the Fascist regime of Mussolini, who by then had slaughtered numerous *partigiani* (partisans) in his home in Sassella, he'd accepted a job offer from a photographic lens manufacturer in eastern Germany and spent three years there with his parents, before returning at the war's end. After they married, they bought out Giuseppina's cousins' share of the vineyard land and began building the house, though construction took many years owing to the post-war recession and a lack of funds.

In the autumn of 2012, I'd returned home to live in Scotland for the first time in over a decade and found work in a tree nursery outside Forres, on the Moray coast. I spent a year there, toying with the idea of calling an end to my years of wandering. But by early summer 2013, the itch had returned – the desire for bigger mountains and a more temperate climate for climbing. I sent my CV to a few schools in mountainous regions, which I'd located using Google Maps, and a week later received a reply from one in a town called Sondrio. The director asked if I could start on Monday, in just four days' time. In the office at work, I returned to Google to remind myself of the town's whereabouts, scribbled out a letter of resignation, and about sixty hours later was on my way. Following my arrival, the first apartment I found sprang a gas leak the day I was due to move in. My boss at the school offered to pay for my hotel while I waited for it to be repaired. In the meantime, his wife told me of an old couple looking to rent the ground floor of their house, more for security than anything else. I went that afternoon and decided to take it before I'd even seen inside.

'My flowers look very peaceful without me bothering them,' Giuseppina calls down, interrupting my daydream. 'Maybe I've never done them much good after all. But they're beautiful, aren't they?'

I nod.

'What day is it today?'

'Tuesday, I think.'

'Maybe Luca will return tomorrow. I miss him.' Luca, Giuseppina's grandson, is a helicopter pilot who works in Apulia. When I spoke to him two days ago, he'd been locked up for ten days inside a seaside hotel, the only guest, waiting for his company to organise a flight home.

I'm still on the terrace when Cristina, Luca's mother, appears. There's no news of when he will return.

'I'm starting to believe this thing was sent by God,' she says. 'To mend us, maybe. There can be no other reason.'

65

I tell her about my cousin and she tells me about a colleague in the Morelli Hospital in Sondalo, a few miles down the valley, which is now the centre for treatment of coronavirus cases in the province.

'It's in the hands of God,' she tells me. As a lifelong atheist, these words have never entered my ear without grating on the way in. 'Excuse me – I know you are not Catholic like us.'

'It's okay,' I say.

'When you sit there, on the terrace, who do you pray to?'

'Nobody. I just watch myself. My own thoughts. It's kinda like knocking on the door to see who's home.'

'I see. Well, everyone has to do what they can, I suppose.'

I take my meditation cushion from inside the apartment and sit under the magnolia tree. Cristina had reminded me that my meditation that morning had been short. Climbing, mountaineering and other forms of physical exertion aside, meditation has been my most important coping mechanism since I was diagnosed as Bipolar in my late teens. While no cure to the onset of more serious episodes, it has given me an awareness of the shiftings of my own mood that I wouldn't have without it, which in turn has allowed me to act sooner should I feel any cerebral mischief in the offing. Today's report: partly cloudy with no storms forecast for the foreseeable, but a chance of a more unsettled outlook moving into next week.

I get a voice message from Holly. She has tested positive but sounds optimistic. Her symptoms are mild and the hospital has sent her home to recover.

On my way inside for dinner I see Enzo dropping off some groceries for Giuseppina. One of his friends died today. A guy of fifty-six, no underlying health conditions.

Seven hundred and forty-three dead today. The past few days' downturn in numbers was short-lived. The light at the end of the tunnel's already snuffed out.

Lockdown Day 17

My phone rings at 5 a.m. It's Bob, my best friend from high school, who now works on an oil rig off the coast of Norway.

'Ah, so you're not dead yet,' he says when I answer.

'It's five in the morning.'

'Aye, sorry about that. Started this isolation shit and it ain't going too well. Or maybe it's going a bit too well, depending on how you see it.'

Bob has been borderline OCD since his early teens, with a particular aversion to germs and dust. I can only imagine what the advent of a lethal microbe has done for his mental state.

'What do you mean?'

'I skipped the loo roll and got a bag of coke, bag of weed and 12 litres of Jim Beam. I'm not due back on the rig for six weeks. My girlfriend, Hayley, works in a frickin' hospital so she's barred, and lives 50 miles away anyway and can't get through the police blockades. And none of my frickin' neighbours seem to give one single hoot about there being a frickin' plague underway so I'm turning this place into the Alamo. With a touch of Vegas, too, granted.'

'Sounds like you're doing fine,' I say. 'Got yourself all set up for the long haul ...'

"Course I have. This thing's spreading like wildfire, just like it's supposed to.'

'Eh?'

'Don't tell me you don't think this ain't all just a *liiiiitle* bit too coincidental. I mean, I'm not one for conspiracy theories, but ...'

'I've heard some rumours, yeah, but they all seemed a little far-fetched.'

'About as far-fetched as that phone you're holding in your hand, muppet. The Chinese have been buying up businesses in the UK and everywhere the past few years and their buying's just gone into overdrive. What better time to grow your empire than when the competition's on its knees, interest rates are zero and you're the only one in town with a chequebook? Anyway, I just wanted to, eh, check in, y'know? Make sure you're doin' okay with your, eh, *heid*, and all that.'

'Nowt to worry about. The *heid*'s fine.'

'Grand. Just remember, you made it through six years o' Waid Academy, so you can make it through a few weeks o' this lockdoon business, nae bother.'

He begins to bring me up to speed on news of our old high-school friends but stops abruptly mid-sentence.

'Shite! I gotta go. Looks like Hayley made it through the blockades after all. Listen: you stay alive, hear me? We've got some growing old to do yet. And if your folks need food or anything, just gimme a shout. I'll be along in a flash.'

Bob had been one of the first to notice the change. I was fourteen. Until then, life had been breezy. I did well in school, I was top scorer in the football team, captain of the golf team. I had a group of friends who were more like brothers, and a sister, mother and father who were more like best friends. I spent weekends climbing and hillwalking with Pa and long nights at the local common pretending I was still as interested in impressing my pals with my football skills as I was my female schoolmates, who'd somehow drifted from the margins of my awareness to somewhere approaching dead centre with alarming alacrity.

Then, things started happening. At first, it just seemed like the same exuberance and moodiness I saw in most of the other pubescent teens around me. But soon there were other experiences that I realised were less typical. Even the smallest incitement of stress or excitement made staying calm problematic. Sitting through hour-long lessons became almost impossible. I'd feel ready to explode if I stayed too long indoors, and had to start jogging for an hour or two before school to oust the excess energy that was making me so irritable and wired throughout the day. I'd always been an emotional and sensitive kid – unfortunate and not exceptionally cool for a teenager stuck in a remote corner of Fife between clusters of fishing and mining villages – but these tendencies seemed to amplify tenfold in little more than a three-month period, in a way that couldn't be accounted for, I was sure, by hormonal fluctuations alone. Soon, I was tearing up in English class whenever Mrs McCance was reading us Auden, Larkin, Heaney or Sassoon, grief-stricken by minor tragedies announced in the morning news, and skipping evening footie games with my friends in favour of stargazing sessions on the beach or all-night lopes around the local woods, where all the subtle variations in light now mesmerised me in ways unthinkable just a few months before.

What I later learned were the 'manic' episodes were usually lengthy but, for the most part, almost enjoyable at their outset. I felt invincible, adored and adoring, and somehow huge despite my gangly, beanstalk stature. I'd go for months on end sleeping just a few hours a night, exercising two or three hours a day, taking just a few days to get through piles of schoolwork that ordinarily would take weeks to complete. Then, though, came the inevitable: the summary segue into bouts of the jitters, anxiety, racing thoughts, insomnia, hyper-sensitivity and hyper-self-consciousness, the feeling that I was watching myself but unable to control what I was doing, and the anomalous and often outrageous behaviour I was only able to identify as such when coming down some weeks, even months, down the line.

The switch to 'depressive' phases would be more abrupt. I'd go to bed, usually feeling as though the mania would never end, then wake to find my seemingly inexhaustible reserves of energy suddenly empty and be unable to leave my room, entirely devoid of the will to see anyone or do any of the things that until then had been the mainstays and cornerstones of every happiness I enjoyed in life.

I began to feel very much an interloper in the human experience. Whether through shame or simple disappointment that nobody I knew shared my way of experiencing the world, I dealt with this newfound awareness of my otherness by removing myself from where the otherness might be noticed, avoiding any situation where I thought my secret was likely to be 'exposed' when I was aware that something was 'up' (or 'down') and steadily withdrawing from almost every staple of the life I'd always known.

I skipped school a lot, leaving home early and bypassing the bus stop before anyone else had arrived, then ducking down an overgrown, bramble-ridden lane to make for the local woods, where I'd spend the day reading and hiding out at the bottom of a steep embankment far from the walking paths.

On days when I made it onto the bus, I'd often change my mind about my ability to face the day ahead during the 45-minute journey to the school. When I met up with Bob for our pre-registration smoke and chinwag about the fortunes of our football team, he'd hand me the key to his house and I'd hole up in his living room, reading his John Fante novels and smoking his dad's cigarettes until it was time for the journey home. The terms Bipolar and depression hadn't entered either of our vocabularies by then, but now, looking back, I realise our three-word morning dialogues marked the first time I spoke of my illness to anyone:

'Keys today?'

'Aye.'

At first, we'd both silently acknowledged that it would be a short-term thing, that eventually the old me would win out against whatever had hijacked my moods and behaviour those past months. But it didn't work out that way. After a few more months, he no longer needed to ask if I needed the key. Instead of a once-in-a-while fallback, it became a regular fixture, and by the time we'd graduated high school, almost a year's worth of my formal education had actually taken place between the understorey of a thicket of sycamore trees and a lonely room in a housing estate far from where my friends and peers were doing adolescence the conventional way.

Viktor Frankl, the Austrian neurologist and psychiatrist who survived a Nazi concentration camp, stated that the discovery of purpose was the key to psychological well-being in both good times and bad. There's an echo there of Nietzsche's 'He who has a why to live can bear almost any how' – or, as Aiyla put it yesterday, 'Don't just sit around on your ass. Find something to do!'

Beyond the need to stay alive to prevent heartbreak to my family, I've identified five things that I believe will help to keep me safe and (relatively) sane:

1. *Projects*. My completed projects to date include sewing the holes and broken seams in all of my climbing clothes, organising my climbing cupboard and baking and freezing enough scones to last me a month. My ongoing projects include turning Giuseppina's garden into the most beautiful in all of Valtellina by the end of lockdown, improving my forearm strength by climbing the wall of the house for at least forty-five minutes per day on crimpy (small) holds only, not getting fired despite the difficulty I've found concentrating these past few days, and spending a few hours a day allaying the fears of the worrisome clan members and responding to messages and emails. My future projects are making a deckchair with repurposed materials to replace the one that's shedding fabric on my terrace as I write, finishing a collection of (admittedly crap) poems I started last summer, and finding a way to reattach the stones in the rear wall that have come loose while I've been climbing and added an element of spice to my pre-dinner sessions.

2. *Avoiding social media*. The bile and disinformation have grown exponentially with the number of days since the lockdown began. One of the virus's most noticeable side effects is that it has minted a spanking-new

batch of polymaths (specialising in epidemiology and international relations) out of roughly 50 per cent of the uninfected and made raging keyboard berserkers out of the rest.

3. *Exercising for at least one hour per day.* Jogging in the vines, rowing, climbing, push-ups, sit-ups, burpees, squats.

4. *Acceptance.* Snuffing out any false hope before it takes hold and taking time to pee on whatever premature victory parade I might, in weaker moments, be planning (my first post-quarantine climb, hike, pizza with friends). This house, these walls, this screen: for now, and maybe for many months to come, that's my universe.

5. *Perspective.* Reminding myself as often as possible of the far worse plight of countless others and remembering all the times in the past when I've wished for just such silence, inactivity and days in which I might have time to make an unrushed phone call to my parents, sister or friends, and to simply while away a few hours without subsequent feelings of guilt for having wasted them.

I sit with Giuseppina for morning coffee again. A cold wind is blowing from the east and today she goes back inside as soon as she's finished.

'There will be better days,' she calls as she waves goodbye from the door.

I work for six hours without interruption.

A fine rain is falling by the time I head outside for my pre-dinner climb. Rather than skip a session or risk slipping on the wet rocks on the back wall, I decide to try the smaller wall below my bedroom window, which is sheltered by Giuseppina's balcony and mostly dry. It's about five metres wide and four metres high and composed of 20x10-inch blocks of pale granite. The traverse is easy but I make things more interesting by gradually eliminating more and more holds for my hands and feet. Nevertheless, I stay as low as possible. Everything now is more consequential. Just as touching the handle of a trolley in the supermarket, inadvertently getting too close to another shopper or an unwitting scratch of an itch on your face might result in infection, a sprained ankle or a broken wrist could be disastrous.

On maybe my fifth traverse, the first voice I've heard all day sounds across the barren expanse between my house and the apartment block below the castle.

'*Professore, cosa fai?*' (What are you doing, teacher?)

I see Benedetta, a former student of mine, on her balcony, clutching her cat Sebastian, an overfed and ill-tempered creature that bears a striking resemblance to a 10-kilo sack of potatoes.

'Hey, Benedetta!' I call up the hill. My voice startles me, so incongruous in the silence that I fancy the very walls of the buildings ringed around the enclosure of Giuseppina's vineyard might object. Yesterday, the government tightened restrictions further by raising the fine for breach of quarantine to a maximum of €3,000, and now, it seems, even the few townspeople with authorisation to be outside have chosen to remain indoors.

'Are you climbing?'

'Yeah.'

'But it's raining.'

'It's okay ... I'm under the balcony.'

'You must be careful! If you fall, who's going to find you?'

'Yeah, good point. I'll be careful.'

'I'm going for dinner now. Sebastian says hi.' She waves the cat's paw at me and disappears inside. The town is again a desert.

Lockdown Day 19

I wake shortly after midnight. Did I hear Giuseppina coughing? I can't be sure it wasn't a dream. I try going back to sleep, but no joy. The birds are out and singing, as if their routine has gone haywire due to all this, too. I make coffee and decide to put in a few hours' work to see if that will tire me out.

My sleeplessness is worrying me. If anything's likely to trigger an episode, it's insomnia. My episodes usually begin with a surfeit of energy, then a two- to four-week period in which everything ranges from being just a little bit special to absolutely magical. Each morning I wake to what appears to be a spanking-new, eighth day of the week. Each time it's like a sky with a new set of stars in it, obliterating the memory of all previous to the point that I'm unable to detect the obvious. On my daily rounds, I'm amazed that nobody else seems to know what's going on, what gorgeousness is at play all around them, or how they can go around being so casual, so immune to awe and wonder. Earth is a kaleidoscope, rushing at me with every colour imaginable. Everything is a giant caper of newly minted marvels, its contents rollicking in ecstasy through every sensory pore and ingress. It's all very, very exciting.

As the days progress, however, usually with less and less sleep, a kind of irritation and antsyness takes over, gradually ripening into the mania which manifests in a clusterfuck of every cerebral antagonism imaginable: anxiety, compulsiveness, restlessness, hypertension, delusion, a perverse enchantment with the idea of self-destruction. I jog for hours on end, climb until my fingers bleed, and rock myself through the long nights, all in an effort to exorcise myself of the energy that would otherwise fuel my neural nemeses.

Then, the inevitable ... the flick of some cerebral switch that kills all the lights, silences the static hum and shuts down the power.

It isn't what people think. Not some plunge from humanness to lowliness. Quite the opposite. This is pith and bone of what it means to be human. Down here I meet me, unadulterated. Unsweetened. Undeodorised. Saccharine-free. Additive-free. Devoid of hope and aspiration and any notion that I may be anything other than 85 kilos of atoms thrown together at random and left to float in a wholly uncaring universe. It is a state of seemingly permanent and irrevocable heartbreak. An oubliette without a door.

I miss Aiyla. And my mum and dad and sister. And my friends. And my townspeople, those I would pass and greet or meet at random on my daily rounds. I miss the days when the everyday worries that occupied my attention (my car's temperamental CD player, the rising cost of plane tickets to Istanbul, the fact that my favourite shampoo leaves my scalp feeling a touch dry) were trifles that now, just three weeks on, I struggle to even remember. I miss newsreaders opening their broadcasts with smiles and the papers wasting column inches on frivolities such as football and reality TV. I miss the mosquito-like hum of my neighbour's three-wheel *ape* when he sets off at 5.30 each morning to tend to his goats and don-keys on a small meadow above the town. I miss the cat videos on Facebook. The levity.

Today's the day I would've been flying back to Istanbul to see Aiyla had the universe not opted to intervene.

I'd spent two decades wandering the globe in search of a place to call home and the partner with whom I'd share it. Two months ago, that dream appeared on the verge of becom-ing a reality: I was finally making enough money freelancing to survive and to be able to visit my parents and sister; in Sondrio, I'd found a place in the world that was more perfectly suited to me than any I could have constructed with the stuff of imagination; I had my Bipolar more or less under control; I had Aiyla. Now, I don't know when I'll see my family or Aiyla again and I'm stuck inside a house, running short on meds, with the mountains that constitute my greatest alter-native medicine visible all around me but off-limits and likely to remain so for months.

Quarantine brings a whole new dimension to the long-distance relationship. Thus far, the obstacles to being together have been bureaucratic and professional. Securing a long-term visa for Italy, Turkey or Scotland would mean marriage – something we've mentioned but not discussed with any seriousness just yet – but at least long-term visa restrictions left scope for our romance to flourish through monthly visits, either here or in Istanbul, and the knowledge that we could be together at the drop of a hat. I'd even planned to rent an apart-ment in Istanbul for the full 90-day duration of a single visa this autumn (once the climbing season was over, naturally . . .).

No more coughing upstairs.

The mouse scuttles across the tiles like a drunk after a night out. On his way he casts me a look. I realise I haven't showered in three days or shaved in a week.

'Sorry,' I say, as he scurries into the hole beneath my biscuit cupboard. 'We have a bit of a situation going on.'

I hear Giuseppina upstairs – the staccato padding of her slippered feet around the kitchen. I sit and listen for an hour for more coughs. None. At 9 a.m. I meet her on the terrace for morning coffee.

'You aren't sleeping,' she says, leaning over the banister. 'I saw your light on in the middle of the night.'

'No,' I confess. 'My brain is too active. But I'll be fine.'

'Are you taking your medicine?'

I didn't know she knew. She was away on a week-long break at the thermal spas in Bormio when I had the episode last spring. I got out of hospital before she returned, but Luca was the one who found me on the lawn and called the ambulance. Maybe he felt obliged to tell her.

'Yes,' I said, and feel guilty that I hadn't told her myself. Of all people, I know she'd be the last to be judgemental.

Earlier I counted thirteen remaining pills. I've decided to split them in two and take one half every other day. I've no idea if that will work, but what other option do I have?

'Good boy,' Giuseppina says. 'Just settle your mind, then. This business is not in our control, so we just have to sit tight and hope it leaves us be – just as we do at other times. And if I can help, let me know.'

Once we've finished our coffees she teaches me the names of the flowers she can see from the balcony, pointing out the newly blooming shrubs in the flowerbed below my terrace and the row beneath the wisteria, whose lilac bells are just beginning to show.

'Your illness . . .' she says, when the lesson has finished and we've been standing for some time, leaning against our respective railings, looking out over the garden. 'Is it . . . What is it?'

My heavily pixelated summary does nothing to unfurrow her brow.

'Basically,' I go on, 'my moods fluctuate severely. There are times when I go for weeks on end without sleeping and I'm full of energy and joy and I lose control of myself and what I'm doing, and others when I can't leave my bed and feel very sad all the time.'

She smiles warmly. 'So,' she says, clasping her hands in front of her, 'you're just a little bit . . . nuts?'

'Exactly,' I say.

'Well, you're in good company now. We're all headed that way these days.'

Her phone rings. She returns inside and reappears a minute later.

'Luca came home last night! He's bringing me groceries later. I'll go inside now and make him some polenta.'

Ma calls before bed. She's crying.

'I just miss you and your sister,' she says. 'It feels like something has ripped the cord between us.'

Since I've lived in Italy, Ma's popped over twice a year to visit. She also makes biannual visits to Brooklyn to visit my sister, Cath, and begins decorating for Christmas in October each year, not out of fondness for the occasion itself but because the day she puts up her tree marks the beginning of the countdown to the annual return of her brood.

'Don't say that, Ma. The cord's still there. It always will be. Christ, we've spent more time on video chat these past few weeks than in the entire decade previously.'

'I know, I'm just feeling it a little bit more today. I've been having these little panic attacks in the night. I'll be fine when I get a good sleep. I was doing fine until yesterday. In fact, I was quite content because all this lockdown business meant you weren't out climbing or up in the mountains with all those avalanches and what have you. But now it's getting worse – all I hear on the news is Lombardy, Lombardy, Lombardy, and now New York, too. You and your sister are at the epicentres of both continents.'

'And we're both locked up at home, going nowhere, washing our hands, not touching our faces, keeping our distance from everyone. We're okay.'

'Yes, I know you'll both be very careful, but it's just, well ... it's a little bit different for you, isn't it?'

'Eh? How?'

'Well, it's not just Covid you have to worry about. I was speaking to Jenny Docherty. She was a nurse, you know? Her dog died last month, the poor thing. She said to keep an eye on you because the whole lockdown business is particularly hard for people with mental health problems. Just promise me you'll take extra, extra, extra good care of yourself.'

'I promise, Ma. I promise.'

I sit at the top of the vineyard after Ma's call. It's evening now, and the orange glow of the lantern-like streetlamps on Via Scarpatetti lights up patches of the cobblestone road and shuttered windows. The bark of a dog far below emphasises the silence. The moonlight seems heavy upon the rustic rooftops, making the tiles sag. A whisper of a breeze flutters the flag on the castle. I sit with my back against the wall and watch a couple doing burpees on their lawn outside one of the houses below.

By now, the fear and anger and anxiety that consumed me at the start of the outbreak have passed, substituted by sadness. The town appears to be mourning, the walls and cobbled streets and rooftops darkened by a veil of sorrow.

Nine hundred and sixty-nine died today.

Lockdown Day 20

Saturday again.

I see Luca after my meditation in the garden. He's on the staircase, putting on the mask and gloves he insists on wearing when visiting Giuseppina, and carrying a bag of medication he's picked up for her from the pharmacy.

'How are you doing?' he asks, descending the stairs so I can hear him through the mask.

I shrug and laugh.

'Same as each of the last twenty-one days ... Bored with flashes of batshit-crazy. How are you and the family?'

'Good,' he says. 'We just don't know how to manage the situation with *Nonna*. I mean, she can't leave the house, she needs food and medication and company, but every time we come in here the risk of infecting her increases. They're limiting ventilators to people under sixty-five, too, so if she got it, she'd be toast.'

'Yes,' I say, 'I've had the same thoughts.'

'And I'm worried about you, too.'

'About me?'

'Yeah.'

Luca had sat with me through the night in the hospital and all of the next day. Despite our closeness, and his insistence on checking up on me every few days all these months down the line, I still have feelings of shame, even guilt, speaking about it with him now. These feelings are to the brain what the appendix is to the body – useless, vestigial remnants – and stem, no doubt, from a childhood in a world even less sympathetic to mental health issues than the one we live in now.

'I know. But don't sweat it. I've got things under control, for now. Just make sure your gran's okay.'

'Aren't you lonely?'

'Yeah, a bit. But I have work to keep me busy. And I'm video-chatting with Aiyla and my family every day. And I have meds . . .'

'Okay, good. But there's one other thing.'

'What's that?'

'The climbing. I'm worried you're going to fall. The neighbours are worried you're going to fall. If you do, and you hurt yourself, nobody's gonna have much sympathy for you. You know that, right? In fact, I can almost feel the fuckers willing you to fall just so they can be all righteous about it afterwards. I mean, I don't want to take away your last bit of enjoyment, but I just . . . you know – I wanted you to know that it might ruffle a few feathers. It's always hard for those who don't climb to understand.'

'Shit, yeah.'

I thank him and go up to my apartment.

In my deckchair, I think over what Luca's told me.

I started climbing at the age of five. My dad was, and is, an enthusiast – a fetishist, you could say. His passion for rock puts the dude who built the Taj Mahal for his missus to shame. Throughout the dark ages of my teenage years, however, climbing took a back seat as Tennent's lager and girls assumed priority in the interludes between bouts of my as-yet-unnamed illness.

If anyone had asked me then if I'd ever climb again, I'd probably have said 'no'. There were so many other things to look forward to – facial hair, more exotic lagers, casual sex, a sparkling career in something or other, universal fame (probably) – that I just couldn't see myself dangling on a rope over lumps of rock.

The end of university, by which point I'd finally been diagnosed with Bipolar, ushered me unwillingly into a world falsely advertised, lacking all the vital ingredients of fun and adventure and containing far more objectionable hardships still. It wasn't all lager. Life, it seemed, was a game of diminishing returns. Soon I'd experienced stress, real relationships, real heartbreak and even a few short-lived bouts of poverty. I'd also thrown into the mix a mental breakdown or two and enjoyed my first hospitalisations for manic clinical exhaustion and two more for overdoses.

I squandered a handful of years in academia and teaching on short-term contracts in the UK, Portugal and Sicily, then one summer returned to Scotland, recently separated from a one-and-only who hadn't read the script, on the dole, constantly aware that the symptoms of my Bipolar were getting worse and certain my appetite for existence had run its course.

One night I made my way to the shed at the bottom of my parents' garden, my grandfather's Smith & Wesson revolver in hand, resolved to finish off the job I hadn't quite been able to accomplish with a cocktail of pharmaceuticals.

The world looks a whole lot different with a gun in your mouth. So different that I convinced myself to give things another go; that there might just be another way to negotiate life without the relentless neurochemical maelstrom that is part and parcel of life with Bipolar 1.

I took the gun from my mouth and made a promise to myself: to give life one last chance to prove it could be something other than the shitshow that had led me to that shed. If it didn't, I'd be back to finish the job.

Logic told me that any life worth living would look very different to the one I'd lived those past few years. Since graduating, I'd lived, studied and taught in large cities – Edinburgh, Phoenix, Lisbon, Palermo. It had been a sedentary life, a cerebral life far removed from my active childhood and youth in Scotland.

Then I landed a teaching job in Trieste, on Italy's Adriatic coast.

Within a month of arriving I'd restarted climbing after discovering Val Rosandra, a gorge cut like a mini Grand Canyon through the flinty karst rock where Istria meets Friuli Venezia Giulia and Slovenia meets Italy. I kitted myself out with new climbing shoes, a rope and a self-belay device that let me climb alone.

Soon I was spending whole weekends there. I'd arrive soon after dawn and leave reluctantly at nightfall. On occasion I'd take my tent and kip at the foot of the crags, scaring the shit out of the wild goats who'd plod sleepily into my encampment of a morning when I was boiling water for my coffee or taking a leak on their thoroughfare. Val Rosandra soon became my Neverland, my weekly fugue into what felt like a foretaste of a life that might just be worth living.

I rediscovered feelings from which I'd been estranged since childhood – joy, wonder, awe, enthusiasm for days ahead. More importantly, eight months after arriving, I felt better than I had done in years and hadn't had even a sniff of an episode. I began to suspect that my battle with Bipolar was one I could win simply by changing the arena in which it was fought. When my teaching contract ended, I knew my next move must be to somewhere similar, but where the mountains would be even more accessible and not a weekends-only kind of fix.

In the years after Trieste, I climbed and hiked extensively in the Himalayas, Karakorum, the Rockies, the Alps, the Dolomites and in my native Scotland. In that time, I accrued more and more evidence that climbing and high places had far more healing power than is commonly acknowledged.

Each time I left on a new adventure, my front door became a rabbit hole through which I discovered wonderlands whose topography and features almost instantly triggered a degree of equanimity and self-awareness that I'm unable to attain elsewhere. Focusing all my energies on the next move means there's little scope for my thoughts to wander to the common sources of their distress. (Finding yourself several hundred feet above the nearest landing place on a thin strand of rope, I've found, is a remarkably effective means of prioritising the resources of headspace to those things most deserving of it. One wrong move and you're a goner.) This focus, I've discovered, segues naturally into an enhanced awareness of my mood and the ability to manage it. On each trip, I also know I'm sure to be blessed at some point by a shift in perspective that lets me look afresh at all the struggles and stressors that may have previously sparked an episode and chuckle at their utter insignificance.

By the time I landed in Sondrio, the literature on the mental health benefits of spending time in nature was beginning to accumulate, but I'd already come to know, from my own experience, that the mental clusterfucks that had so blighted my youth and early adulthood found their kryptonite in the form of altitude, fresh air, empty landscapes and the devotion of all energies to the task in hand – a far simpler formula than trial-and-erroring through various life-sapping pharmaceuticals. In Sondrio I've managed to find a workable balance between climbing and professional obligations, with my freelance schedule allowing me to squeeze in around four climbs per week, either at local crags or in the high mountains. I exercise every day, but climbing is now an immovable fixture at the top of my weekly list of non-negotiables – as imperative as any medication, therapy or coping strategy.

But how I might explain all this to my surrogate family members and neighbours is beyond me. The idea of surrendering that privacy and this last liberty to the heat of peer pressure annoys me, but they have a point – the last thing the hospital needs is people coming in with easily avoided injuries. But I also know that my need to stay healthy of mind mitigates the community's interest in all of its uninfected members, myself included, easing the strain on the hospitals by ensuring we stay healthy of body – as does my decision to never climb high enough on either of the traverses to do myself much more damage than a sprain.

I decide to leave the decision over whether I should

continue to Giuseppina, half-suspecting that maybe her gentility and courteousness has led her to ask Luca to have a quiet word on her behalf. If that's the case, and she's been made to feel at all nervous, I'll have to stop.

I catch her later that afternoon, after Luca has returned home. I'm sitting under the staircase, on my decomposing deckchair, doing some prep for tomorrow's work on my laptop, when she appears on the steps with a watering can.

'Thank you, Kieran,' she says. 'The garden's looking better now than it has in years. The gardener's going to be mightily jealous when this all finishes and he comes back to see it!'

'You're welcome!' I say.

I leave my seat and step back to make way for her to pass across my terrace into the garden.

'I wanted to ask you,' I say, while she's still making her way down. 'Are you still okay with me climbing? The neighbours aren't too happy, apparently.'

'Why wouldn't they be? We need these things. Enjoyment, I mean. Otherwise it becomes only misery.'

'They're afraid I'll fall. With the hospitals overstretched . . .'

'Pfffft! They could say the same about me with my watering can! Now, you listen . . .'

She climbs down another few steps and places the can on the ground.

'We built this house as a sanctuary for our family. For us and for generations to come. You are our family now and you may do within this property whatever you please.'

I feel such an urge to hug and kiss her that I have to take another step back.

'Luca is a good boy. He is concerned for you, and I'm proud

87

to have a grandson with such a big heart. He's just like his grand-father, God bless him. But you have to live your life as well as you can within whatever restrictions there may be – money, religion, politics, viruses, and even nosy neighbours. Now go ... Get your shoes on and show them you're not scared!'

I do as I am told. During my regular quota of pre-dinner traverses, I even wave, mid-climb, to one neighbour who appears on his balcony. He waves back and laughs, shaking his head. I think I love him.

Later, I sit and watch the dimming sky. The smell of dinners being cooked in the surrounding houses delivers a punch of homesickness. I picture all the families sitting at tables together and can't help but imagine Ma and Pa, with their trays on their laps, sitting in the living room watching the evening news. Longer periods have passed in which I haven't seen them, but the uncertainty as to when I'll see them again is dizzying.

I read the news before bed. A 29-year-old committed suicide near Torino after the lack of financial help from the government saw his business collapse. Albania has sent thirty doctors to help in Italian hospitals. Italians are appealing to Germany to remember their forgiveness of German war debt in 1953 and provide the assistance it has thus far refused. Boris Johnson isn't dead.

Another 756 Italians are.

Lockdown Day 22

Another letter in the post. Another bill. Another trip to the bank.

I thought the mail service was being suspended? As I stroll

down Via Scarpatetti, I feel myself lumbering over the cobblestone cubes like a novice to bipedalism. The sound of my feet seems a profanity in the silence. It's been so long since I walked here that my senses can barely keep up with the novelty of so many things so long unseen, unsmelt and unheard. It's as if each sense has become heightened in the absence of stimuli. I hear the odd noise from the windows above – a television, plates in a sink, the murmur of voices, shutters opening. The smell of cigarette smoke, rubbish bins stacked below the archway halfway down, and the sweetness of last night's rain warming in a timid morning sun all contribute to the feast, a veritable smorgasbord of the sensuous.

I pass no one until I reach the bell-tower square, where I see a figure scuttling through the doors of the city-council office. In Piazza Garibaldi, the central square, a police car is parked outside the entrance to the bank and an orderly line of five people at two- or three-metre intervals is waiting, stretching back to the statue of the man himself in the centre. At this time of year, the cafés around the square's periphery are normally filled with people on breaks from work, drinking coffee or Aperol spritz and eating *brioche* in daily celebration of the end of their winter hibernation. Today the square is deserted, the cafés locked and boarded, the white, pink and yellow stone of the *palazzi* more sombre than in even the bleakest days of winter.

I take my place in the queue behind an elderly couple. A policeman is checking the self-certification documents of those at the front of the queue, and a security guard is restricting entrance to one person at a time.

I hear the click of heels behind me. The clicks grow louder until I find a woman beside me, at least a metre closer than the two-metre stipulation. I scuttle a few steps forward, and then another to the side to ensure I don't get too close to the elderly couple in front. The woman promptly steps into the unoccupied space, forcing me to take another sideways step into the no man's land flanking the queue.

The Italians' inability to do queues is about equal to British people's fury should anyone skip them or flout queuing conventions. Their collective non-compliance to the formality of standing in a straight line is as ingrained as the language, and something that must be accepted and tolerated no less than their demand that we drive on the right-hand side of the road.

'Have you been waiting long?' the high-heeled lady asks the elderly couple, reaching out with a hand.

I restrain myself.

'Please,' says the man, shrugging off her hand, 'respect the distance. We've been here about ten minutes. They're taking one at a time.'

The woman sighs and lights a cigarette. She continues to hover between me and the old couple. The old couple shuffle forward as the security guard ushers the first in line inside. I move to reclaim my place in the queue. No sooner have I done so than the lady is breathing down my neck, her cigarette smoke passing over my shoulders. I turn to give her a death stare, but she's on the move again before it hits its target, approaching the old couple once more.

'You have to move forward,' she tells them, saltily, 'otherwise they won't see you and won't let you in.'

'We know the system,' the man says, shielding his wife behind him. 'Now please ...' He takes a short step forward and waves the woman away.

She humours him with a half-step back. When finished with her cigarette, she tosses the stub onto the stone paving and struts to the entrance to speak to the guard. I can't hear what she says but she soon returns, visibly flustered. By now there is another client waiting in line behind me but the lady resumes her place by my side and pulls out her phone. I turn to face her and speak in as calm and measured a voice as I can.

'The two metres mentioned in the *decreto* is not a recommendation,' I tell her, 'but a law. Either walk two or get thrown five. Do you understand?'

She backs up a few steps and begins cursing volubly. The old man in front of me turns and smiles.

'Thank you,' he says.

'My pleasure.'

I notice I'm shaking as the guard waves me through the doors. I'm guided to the first desk, where I'm asked to fill out a form for statistical data analysis. After doing so, I rub my hands down with sanitiser before being ushered to a second desk, where I briefly chat with another clerk, who guides me to a third desk on the other side of the room. There I wait for ten minutes before one of the masked trio of workers arrives at their computer. There are two more forms. I take out my sanitiser again, then, realising I'd grabbed the bottle immediately after using the pen on the counter to fill out the forms, I sanitise my sanitiser. The clerk's eyes suggest he's smiling beneath his mask.

'Aren't you the Scottish teacher?' he asks. 'The one who wears the kilt?'

I smile and nod. For three years I taught two groups of bank employees and a couple of the company directors. On occasion, I'd try to break the monotony of our 'Financial English' lessons with a change of clothes.

'I haven't seen you in years. Don't you teach any more?'

'I stopped a few years ago. I'm freelance now. I wanted more freedom to visit my family.'

'Shit!' he says. 'Then why didn't you go back to Scotland before this happened?'

'I have a feeling I might be safer here.'

'Maybe. Your new prime minister makes even Berlusconi look good.'

The security guard clears his throat behind us and nods towards the line of people waiting by the door.

By 5 p.m. the rain has stopped and I go into the garden. Giuseppina comes to join me while I'm weeding around the daffodils that came into flower overnight. She waves to me as she enters the garden and takes a trowel to plant some flowers that her daughter, Monica, brought with her groceries the other day. As I continue weeding along the base of the roadside wall, I see her in the corner of my eye, inspecting a flowerbed in the far corner. I carry on weeding. While I'm crouched over, trying to dig out the roots of a particularly stubborn, prickly sprig at the base of the wall with a trowel, I feel her hand on my head.

'Don't overexert yourself, *ragazzo*,' she says, ruffling my hair. 'If it won't come, it won't come.'

It is the first time I've been touched by another human in twenty-three days.

Before dinner I head outside again to put in an hour on the walls. Another light shower has wetted the rear garden wall so I content myself with the shorter but slightly trickier facade of the house under Giuseppina's balcony. By now I know each move by heart and I imagine I'll soon be able to complete the five-metre traverse with my eyes closed and by feel alone.

I decide against putting my memory to the test right now but up the stakes slightly by using only holds I've never used before and lengthening the route. I start below my living room, forcing myself into a bridging movement in the 90-degree corner to reach the east-facing wall of my bedroom, then around a 270-degree corner to return to the gable wall. While approaching the latter, I spot a large gap between two of the granite blocks. It looks ready-made for a fist- or finger-jam, a technique employed in climbing on long, vertical fissures that involves inserting the hand into the crack and then balling the fist until it is locked in place. As I close my fist in the gap, a bolt of pain shoots through the back of my hand. I know instantly what has happened. With my smarting hand hanging by my side, I pull up with my other hand and glance into the hole, where my tiny black assailant is frozen in place, his palps and stinger still braced for defence. My hand has doubled in size by the time I reach the bathroom to disinfect the wound, which continues to ache almost exquisitely throughout dinner and long into the night. While I'm lying in bed, I remember some of the symptoms associated with scorpion stings, which I'd googled after discovering the first of the fifty or so of the critters that I've found in my apartment since I first moved here: fever, body aches, dryness in the throat, difficulty swallowing. All very Covid-like.

The next few days are going to be swell.

Lockdown Day 23

My hand is a balloon. The throbbing wakes me at 4 a.m. and I stumble into the kitchen for coffee and to inspect the damage. My fingers are like oversized carrots and my entire hand an unhappy shade of plum. Going to the hospital is not an option, so I decide to give it time.

Holly calls at 6 a.m. I sent her a picture of my hand last night.

'Okay,' she says. 'Have you got a fever?'

'Nope.'

'Are you having difficulty breathing?'

'Nope.'

'Swallowing?'

'Nope.'

'Has the swelling increased since last night?'

I pull up the sleeve of my shirt and discover that the swelling has migrated halfway up my forearm.

'Yeah, I think so.'

'Let me see it,' she says.

I hold the hand to the phone.

'Sweet Jesus,' she says. 'What a mess.'

'It'll be okay. It's just like a bad bee sting.'

She purses her lips and gives them a pensive wiggle.

'Okay, so here's what you need to do ...'

At some point while she's speaking I notice the pallor and gauntness in her face and remember how the only reason she hadn't been taken into intensive care last week was because she'd refused to burden the already overburdened hospital unless absolutely necessary ('Very British of me, eh?'). She's also far from out of the woods. Troubling her with something as trivial as a sting from a scorpion the size of an overweight caterpillar seems embarrassing. Her rasping cough only confirms the point.

'Sweet Jesus,' I say.

'Oh, that's nothing. This time last week you probably could have heard me without the phone.'

She goes on to tell me that the hospital was diagnosing patients almost exclusively with blood tests owing to the lack of swabs. A high white-cell count would reveal pneumonia, tuberculosis or a regular fever, whereas a low count meant a viral infection, i.e. coronavirus. She had the latter. Her treatment, she tells me, consisted solely of high-dosage shots of vitamin C, something that thus far has proven to be the most effective means of treating patients prior to intubation.

'I don't understand why this isn't all over the news,' I say, thinking of the dozens of reports I've read proclaiming that no vaccine, antibody or therapeutic will be ready for several months.

'Because big pharma wouldn't want to miss out on their payday, of course. Don't tell me you were naive enough to think that the way of the world would change just because of a little pandemic? Wait . . .'

My phone pings with two new messages.

'I just sent you the numbers of two doctor friends. I called them this morning and they say they'd be happy to pay a home visit if need be.'

'Holly, they can't.'

'Risky, I know, but don't be so bloody British. If someone offers their help, take it.'

I monitor my hand throughout the day, re-marking where

the swelling ends with a pen every few hours, as Holly has recommended. It doesn't seem to be getting any worse.

I wrap the hand in a soaked tea towel and sit down to work.

Dad calls in the afternoon.

'Guess what I did this morning?' he says, unnaturally chipper.

'I'm hoping the answer is either jack shit or taking down Aunty Jane's artwork from the dining room.'

'I did the chain walk.'

The chain walk is a via ferrata-like climbing–hiking hybrid route near my parents' home, where giant fixed chains thread a slightly perilous path over and around a half-mile stretch of sea cliffs. It's one of my favourite spots in the world, but also one where dozens of accidents occur each year.

'Dad, what the—?'

'Don't worry, now. It was perfectly safe. I left at three in the morning and was home again in time for breakfast. Didn't see a single soul until I was back in the garden and opening the door.'

'That wasn't the concern. What if you'd fallen or slipped, or had another HM?'

In the past few years, Dad's had a handful of hemiplegic migraines, the second of them resulting in him being air-lifted off a mountainside in the Highlands, losing his driving licence, and being forced into a six-month break from walking and climbing.

'I must have done that thing five hundred times and I haven't fallen once. Besides, bugger it – they can't take away all our freedoms.'

It's very easy to imagine myself speaking the same words.

'I miss you, laddie,' he says. 'The only thing that would

have made this morning better would have been you being there with me. The snowdrops are coming. And the sand-pipers were out in their droves. And I saw two herons in the burn by Shell Bay. A cold easterly but blue skies all the way.'

'I miss you too, *Faither.*'

Soon after lunchtime I hear Giuseppina talking upstairs. When she forgets to put in her hearing aid, her phone voice can be heard by anyone within a 200-metre radius. She's speaking to her bestie, Antonella, who lives in the neigh-bouring *comune* of Triangia, a few miles away on the slopes of Monte Rolla. They've spent nearly every day together since Domenico's death. In the past year, I've caught the pair of them taking drives in Valmalenco, walking on the third-tier path above the vineyards (some 400 vertical metres above the town) and gossiping like teenagers in Portec, the little cave-like bar on Via Scarpatetti, but I haven't seen Antonella's 1973 Fiat Special parked on the hill outside the house since the ban on leaving your *comune* of residence.

Half an hour later, I see Giuseppina in the garden while I'm stretching my legs on the top tier of the lawn.

'I was on the phone to Antonella!' she tells me, climbing down the stairs in her slippers, thin beige slacks and a cardigan that seems far too flimsy for the chilly northerly blowing down from Valmalenco and Switzerland.

'She's well. She said I should walk in the garden, to make good use of what I have. She has no garden so she's doing laps of her kitchen table. Ha! Shall we do some gardening?'

I have a deadline at 6 p.m. but decide there's time and fetch my gloves, more to hide my hand than anything else.

We decide on trying to regrow the grass on the bare patches beneath the magnolia.

'They're an eyesore,' she says. 'They never recovered from that very dry year we had – do you remember? It must have been five years ago. Gosh, you've been with me for such a long time.'

'I remember. I remember the heat – sitting out on the terrace with Domenico in our shorts, praying for wind and rain.'

'Ah, yes. I wonder what my Domenico would make of all this. He was a good man. A kind man.'

'He was the best.'

He *was* the best. Every time someone came to visit me, I'd invariably find a €50 note slipped under my door on the first morning with a note attached – *'per birra e pizza'* ('for beer and pizza'). One summer I went to visit him and Giuseppina at the caravan they were staying in in Poschiavo and he spent the day giving me a tour of the neighbouring villages on his electric bike and introducing me to the locals. Another time, he'd been cycling down by the river and spotted me coming out of a café with my colleagues. He slammed on his brakes in the middle of the road and held up a line of fifteen or so cars for five minutes while introducing himself to everyone and inviting them to dinner. In the last few months before he died, filled with morphine, he'd still call over the balcony whenever he saw me in the garden and invite me up for snacks and the cans of Coca-Cola he bought specially to accommodate my teetotalism.

'Anyway, before I get myself teary, let's get those seeds and figure out what to do with them.'

I fetch the bag from the shed behind the house, but the instructions have faded and are no longer legible.

'Don't worry,' I say. 'We can check Google.'

'This Google does everything these days. Soon I imagine it will jump out of the phone and plant seeds for us.'

Just then, Enzo, her son-in-law, appears at the gate with a tray of strawberries and oranges.

'Vitamin C delivery!' he calls across the garden. His expression changes as Giuseppina emerges from behind the Japanese maple.

'What are you doing out here dressed like that? Get inside and get a jacket on! And some proper shoes! There's a wind blowing directly from Siberia!'

Giuseppina slants her eyes towards me.

'This is when I should pretend I haven't turned on my hearing aid,' she says. Then, turning to Enzo: 'Very well.'

She shuffles back across the grass and up the stairs like a scolded schoolgirl.

While she's inside I show Enzo my hand.

'Like a melon and five sausages,' he says. 'Don't worry. People can die from the stings but you're too big. If you start having trouble breathing, though, give me a call and I'll get you a doctor.'

'Will it be so easy?'

'Of course. This is Italy – you can do things the formal way and spend half your life waiting, or do them the informal way and have them taken care of "like that". There are two Italys – the one you see and the one you don't.'

'I like the informal.'

'Of course you do. The formal way is for foreigners and bankers. You've been here long enough to consider yourself a local and I'd be surprised if you even have a bank account.'

At 6 p.m. I sink to a new level of absurdity, returning to

the garden with a wet tea towel wrapped around my hand for my nightly climbing session.

Aiyla calls while I'm on the wall, which I've taken to calling the 'Dusk Wall' in honour of Yosemite National Park's Dawn Wall and because it captures the last rays of the sun before it dips below Castel Masegra and the valley floods with the violet gloaming.

'If the scorpion gets your other hand this time, does that mean you'll take a break?'

'Unlikely.'

'You know, I'm writing an article on internet addiction for a journal. I can see parallels.'

'There's a difference. Those addicts form addictions to escape *from* reality. This is an escape *into* reality.'

'Explain.'

'Well, it's very tangible. The rock. And your body. We glaze over so many things we see every day, making our experience very superficial. When you're climbing, that isn't an option. You have to be present and focused. It's the opposite of the only other alternatives right now: staring at my phone or laptop screen, which are both very virtual, voyeuristic, vicarious.'

'Hmmm, that makes sense,' she says. 'Okay, so, don't get too excited, but maybe I'll give it a try. Next time you come.'

This is big. A game-changer, maybe. Since we first met, the knowledge of how different we are as people has always hung in the background. Aiyla is light and carefree, a clean-freak, a lover of fashion and architecture, and can spend entire weekends in shopping malls. I am dark and brooding, more laissez-faire about hygiene and orderliness, and dress in a mix of hand-me-downs and more-functional-than-fashionable climbing threads; I consider mountain huts and tents the apotheosis of desirable residences, and the only non-perishable goods I've bought in the past decade have been from the same climbing store. Our relationship has flourished because of our differences, but I always feared a point would come where our incompatibility would be exposed.

'I'd love that,' I say.

'Do you think the sting will give you superhuman powers, like Spider-Man?'

'You mean *more* superhuman powers, right?'

'Since when have crazy stubbornness and flatulence been considered superhuman powers?'

Before we hang up she suggests a new name for the wall. No. 3 Via Aurelio Fracassetti is now home to two named climbing areas: the Dusk Wall and the Scorpion Wall.

Lockdown Day 24

Wednesday.

I turn on my phone for my daily dose of the absurd.

Turkmenistan has banned its media from using the word 'coronavirus'; Donald Trump's 'hoax' is now a recognised formidable foe likely to kill in the region of 200,000 Americans; regional UK police departments are using creative interpretations of the PM's lockdown decree, dyeing pools in popular wild swimming spots black to put off swimmers, filming walkers with drones and fining shoppers for buying non-essential provisions like Easter eggs; police in Kenya have shot and killed a 13-year-old on his balcony while enforcing curfew, fired teargas at commuters and beat others with batons; migrant workers in Delhi are being sprayed with a bleaching agent to disinfect them before they return to their home provinces; Paraguayan officers are forcing quarantine violators to do star jumps and threatening them with tasers; Hungary has introduced jail terms for spreading misinformation about the virus.

Here in Italy, it's been discovered that a woman who fled Lombardy on 9 March brought the virus to Naples, resulting in a mob of angry protesters baying for blood outside her home; the government warns that social-distancing measures will be in place long after the end of quarantine, awards €600 each to both freelance workers and the estimated 4 million employed in under-the-table jobs and allows parents to walk their children; meanwhile, 'to feed the pigeons', 'to walk the cat' and 'love' are just a few of the reasons cited for leaving home on official self-certification documents of those stopped by the police.

The swelling in my hand has gone down.

Over breakfast I remember the dream I had in my fitful hour or so of sleep. It started out as a recreation of my last real climb before lockdown. In late November, I set off with Gaia, a friend from Lissone, to climb a multi-pitch route of some 300 metres in Val di Mello, an offshoot valley a few miles north-west of Sondrio that's internationally renowned as a climber's Mecca. On the phone beforehand, she told me she'd been training in the months since I last saw her. She'd learned how to climb multi-pitch with her new boyfriend and was desperate to try a big route. With this information, I'd decided on a climb called 'L'Albero delle Pere', a testy but perfectly doable route on the valley's north side.

We set off early and arrived at the foot of the climb at around 9 a.m., after a short hike. They call the valley 'The Yosemite of Europe'. Huge granite monoliths abbreviate the sky in all directions. Between them, cascading waterfalls cut through banks of old-growth forest. On the valley floor, a scattering of stone *baite* (mountain dwellings) half hidden among the trees are like crumbs spilled by the giant heads of the peaks above.

'They're fucking huge,' Gaia says as we hiked up the flanks of the river that splits the valley, her eyes trained upward on the northern domes of Monte Qualido and Scoglio della Metamorfosi.

'Yup.'

It was unseasonably warm. As we geared up at the foot of the climb, the thick bank of cloud that hung over the valley, impaled on the jagged summit of Monte Disgrazia to the east, began to part, boding well for the day ahead. Our progress was hampered at first by a rain shower, then by difficult route-finding and an overhanging roof that I was slow to negotiate. Gaia remained stuck beneath the roof for over three hours. When she finally made it, there was still plenty of daylight left so we decided to push on to the top, from where we'd be able to walk back down to the valley on a path descending from the hanging valley to the west. However, another testy pitch slowed us down further, and halfway up the next, after losing another hour trying to find the route, we decided to abseil down rather than risk trying to climb the final two pitches in the dark.

The sun had dropped below the peaks to my left by the time I recovered my gear and began climbing back down to Gaia, who was belaying me from a narrow ledge below. When I finally reached her, we were in almost complete darkness and quickly prepared our equipment for the abseil.

I told Gaia to take out her head torch.

'I left it in the car,' she replied.

The alarm on her face reminded me of the need to appear as calm as possible, despite the panic brewing in my chest.

'It's okay. Whoever goes first can use my head torch, the second can set themselves up with their phone light.'

A tear glided over her cheek in the light from my head torch.

'Wait – what's wrong?' I asked.

'I didn't tell you. I haven't learned to abseil, not properly. The routes I did with my boyfriend were walk-off, so there was no need. I learned the basics but now I can't remember.'

'Shit. Okay, don't worry.'

'Should we phone for help?'

'There isn't any signal here. Anyway, it's okay. I'll just set up your abseil for you and you can go first.'

'No! *Please* – I can't do that. Just show me how it's done and I'll follow you down.'

'What if I lower you?'

'No, please. I don't want to go first. Even with the head torch it's terrifying.'

The night was strangely warm. I considered making a bivouac on the ledge, but didn't want to risk the temperature dropping during the night.

I spent another hour giving Gaia a refresher course on abseiling, making her repeat the set-up six or seven times to make sure she had it down before setting off myself.

I completed the first abseil and anchored myself into the next belay point, a collection of brightly coloured slings tied through a duo of old pitons jammed into cracks in the rock. I gave three strong tugs on the rope to signal to Gaia to follow. She didn't. The rope remained limp and motionless. I tried calling, but there was no reply. It was an hour before I finally felt movement in the rope and another half-hour before I saw her emerge from the overhang above me. As I was helping to tie her into the anchor, I knocked my head against her side. Before I knew what had happened, I saw a strobe of light spinning down the cliff and landing some 200 metres below, then go out.

'Fuck.'

'Fuck.'

Now we had only our phones.

I set off on the next abseil. With both hands occupied with the ropework, I was dependent on the light of the moon to find my way and locate the next anchor. I backed myself onto the edge of a rounded ledge, a feature I couldn't remember passing on the way up. The spurts of vegetation between the rocks were perfectly still. The moon appeared absurdly big in the pocket of sky between the pearl-white bust of Monte Disgrazia's upper slopes and a bank of wispy cloud above. My breath was the only sound. With my feet pressed against the last block of visible rock, I looked down. There was nothing – only a darkness so thick it almost seemed it would catch me if I were to let go. I knew the valley floor was some 1,000 feet below, but from here it seemed as though the void beneath me might continue for ever. I had one last moment of doubt before leaving. The section of the route still below us, I remembered, had climbed the face diagonally, but gravity dictated that our descent would be vertical, meaning we wouldn't be able to use the same anchors that we'd used on the ascent for the remaining abseils after this one. I knew there were routes parallel to ours with other anchors, but didn't know if I'd be able to find them without my head torch, nor if our ropes would be long enough to reach them.

'I'll give you a tug when I'm down there,' I said to Gaia, then began my descent.

Just a few metres down, I found myself hanging over the cliff face in empty space. The silence was absolute, the shuffle of my hands on the rope only emphasising the complete absence of any other sound. The darkness of the inky night sky was so dense that I felt I could grab hold of it. Below me, in the distance, I saw a few lights from the *baite* on the valley floor. Some 20 metres down I locked off my safety and let myself dangle in my harness to take it all in.

I must have been hanging in place for fifteen minutes before Gaia called from above.

'Is everything okay?'

'Yeah!' I called back. I'd been so immersed in the exquisiteness of the moment that I'd almost forgotten the context, the shitshow that preceded it and, to all appearances, was due to continue for some time. 'I'm just finding the route.'

I found the anchor.

Gaia and I finally made it down to the valley floor at 3 a.m., dehydrated and exhausted. In the dream, however, I remained on the rope, dangling in space, snug in the womb-like embrace of the darkness and emptiness. I understood I would stay there for ever and, rather than panic or despair, felt myself suffused with an all-encompassing warmth and peace the like of which I've never known. It seemed to transfer from the me in the dream into the me that was sleeping in my bed. When I woke, I woke smiling. The tension permeating my body these past few weeks had vanished, along with the anxiety that has been my loyal bedmate each night since I left Istanbul. I tried to go back to sleep, back to the sheltering pocket of sky high on the granite walls above Val di Mello, but then I remembered . . .

Giuseppina has visitors – her daughter Monica and grand-daughter Anna, I think – so I have no excuse for putting off the backlog of work that's stacking up in the 'Unread' section of my inbox. I see her only in the late afternoon, when I stumble into the garden to read my book, dazed from a full day in front of my computer.

'There you are,' she says. 'Where have you been today?'

She's kneeling in front of the clusters of peonies and lobelia we planted yesterday, dropping pellets of fertiliser around them with all the care of a cake-maker.

'Chi non lavora, non mangia,' I tell her (He who doesn't work, doesn't eat) with a shrug, and grab the shears to start trimming around the perimeter walls.

'No, put those down. Today you should rest. Come, we can sit together on the grass. You sit on the middle tier; I'll sit on the top one. That way we'll be far enough apart but I'll still be able to hear you.'

We pull our deckchairs onto the lawn and align them with the gap between the maple and a hydrangea.

As we sit, I realise there's very little to talk about, something I've encountered in the past few days when calling Aiyla, my sister and my parents. It's becoming difficult to remember what we talked about before the virus, and talk of anything else is always tinged with the feel of an exercise in avoidance.

As we sit, I'm slapped with a dose of the surreal. I think of all the social media posts in which people have shared photos of their experiences in lockdown – families, couples, climber friends scaling bookcases and stairwells as housemates or pets look on. For the first time, I realise that I'm in quarantine with a 90-year-old Italian widow, a long way from Fife.

'Your parents,' she says, 'do they have a garden?'

'A small one. My father is out there almost every day doing something.'

'I imagine it's all nice and green. That's what I've always imagined about those places – how green they must be. That's the one thing we don't have here – that and the sea. Tell me again about your little village.'

'Well, it's tiny. When I was young, there were maybe only 400 people. Now it's maybe closer to a thousand. There's one shop, one bar and a post office. It's surrounded by fields and forests on one side and the sea on the other. I can hear the waves from my bedroom window at night, when it's quiet. When I visit in the summer, I walk down to the beach in my bare feet and take a dip if it's warm enough. There's a path that goes all along the coastline for miles and miles. On the way you pass through all these old fishing villages with ancient harbours and brightly painted houses. We never appreciated it when we were young but now each time I'm back it's wonderful . . . like discovering a new land every time.'

'And what do the people do?'

'All kinds of things. Once upon a time it was a fishing village, I suppose, but the industry collapsed about twenty years ago. Now there's no work, so people travel to the cities, like Edinburgh or Dundee.'

'Like Milan, here. I lost my girls for years when they went to the university and then started working.'

She pulls a purple leaf from a branch of the hydrangea and crushes it in her fingers.

'What are the chances,' she says, shaking her head, 'of a lad from a small village up there coming to live here, halfway around the world. I'd never have imagined it.'

'I got lucky,' I tell her.

'No, we were the lucky ones. And your girl is a lucky one too. You will make her a good husband if she's smart. How is she doing? Is she well?'

I spoke to Aiyla this morning. She called at 6 a.m., unslept, caked in flour and margarine from her latest baking experiment in her mother's kitchen.

'Yes,' I say. 'She's with her family. They're like us – just waiting for all this to pass.'

'It's high time you and Luca found yourselves wives,' she says. 'By your age I'd had all three of my daughters. Domenico and I had been together for years. Do you think she will be the one?'

'It's hard to say.'

'It shouldn't be. In fact, it's very simple. You must ask yourself something: is she the one you want to have beside you at your deathbed when that time comes? If so, you have your answer.'

We sit for another half an hour before either of us speaks again. The sun is high over the peaks of the Orobie. Squeals of kids' laughter come from a garden on the hill behind us. A lawnmower hums in the distance, temporarily obscuring the sound of the sirens. It could be any other day in any other year.

'What is the book?' Giuseppina asks, pointing at the paperback in my lap.

It's an anthology of Tennyson, a book I've carried every-where since I was a teenager. I flash her the cover, a portrait of the bearded poet in dignified pose.

She gives an approving nod.

'Maybe you could read something to me.'

'It's in English.'

'No matter. You can translate for me afterwards.'

I read her 'Ulysses'. While I'm reading she closes her eyes and nods in time with the completion of each line.

'What does it speak of?' she asks, as soon as I've finished.

'It's about an old man, Ulysses, who returns to domestic life after years of travelling and adventure. He speaks of his desire to go exploring again, despite his age.'

'Ha! Now I understand why you like it! And how does he resolve his problem?'

'He doesn't, really. It's more like a battle cry, a pledge to use himself up until his very last day, to continue adventuring.'

'And what about you? Will you continue adventuring after this?'

'I don't know.'

In my late twenties and early thirties, I spent five or six years wandering the globe, living in my tent, communes, and short-lease apartments where I never stayed long enough to bother buying any more suitable sleeping paraphernalia than my sleeping bag. I was, I guess, what you'd call a 'spiritual seeker'. I spent months in sweat lodges in the American Southwest and Croatia, joined a cult-like spiritual group in the north of Scotland, lived in a monastery for a few months in the Himalayas and dug a grave on a hillside in Slovenia and spent the night inside it, contemplating death, on the counsel of a shaman who'd also convinced me to spend one day every week for a year interrogating an unexceptional rowan tree in a remote wood on the Italian–Slovenian border.

At that time, I think I believed that the movement itself was a form of treatment, as if there could be some kind of geographical solution to my problems. Like they could be outrun, or I'd land somewhere and they just wouldn't be there any more. But that never really happened. And the main catalyst, I suppose, was denial. Shame, even. Whenever I'd been anywhere too long and felt on the brink of becoming too close or attached to people, I moved on before they could find out. It was an act of self-preservation, pre-emption. My episodes were destructive enough, but their aftermaths were soul-destroying. I'd go into them with friends, partners, jobs and dreams, and come out of them with nothing. To spare myself that agony, and to keep my secret a secret, I just jumped ship. It's still maybe my biggest fear – that I'll lose everything and be powerless to stop it. Even though my experiences in Sondrio thus far suggest I might have finally turned a corner, the condition's constant evolution and penchant for untimely curveballs and tits-up reversals of fortune mean I've never felt safe enough to allow myself the luxury of planning too far ahead.

'I think this is a modern disease, this not knowing,' Giuseppina says. 'It's the same with my granddaughters. I ask them anything and they don't know. When we were young, you knew everything. There were limitations in that, of course, but there was a beauty in it too. A freedom, even. We made the most of things with the resources that were at our disposal and within the limitations imposed by things outside our control. Simple.'

'This Brexit business has made it more difficult. I'm not a citizen. And my girlfriend is Turkish, not European. And even before this virus I worried about my parents every day. They're getting old and I know that my sister and I are the main source of happiness in their lives – sometimes it feels wrong to deprive them of that happiness for all but a few weeks every year.'

'The answers will come to you, I'm sure. But you would be missed if you were ever to leave here. Just look at yourself – you seem to belong to the landscape more than people born and bred here. You're a Valtellinese.'

Lockdown Day 25

I wake at 2 a.m. to the sound of rustling outside my window. Through a gap in the shutter I see silken streams of moonlight draped over the vines but not the source of the disturbance. I put on my dressing gown and fumble through the dark to the kitchen window. There, I see a fox sniffing at the cellar door. He lunges towards it, as if trying to shoulder-barge it open, but scampers off when I turn on the kitchen light.

I try to get back to sleep but notice my phone flashing with an incoming call. It's a client in the US who, despite our four-year association, hasn't grasped the concept of differing time zones.

'I was wondering,' she says, 'how many assignments do you think you can take on this month?'

'I should—' I begin, before she interrupts.

'Well, I was thinking, with this lockdown and all, maybe you could handle a few more?'

'Yeah,' I say, still too sleepy to consider the consequences. 'No problem.'

'Awesome. I'll send them over ay-sap.'

They've arrived by the time I've made coffee and taken my seat at the window. There are twenty of them, a 100 per cent increase on my usual monthly total. Instinctively, my mind begins doing the maths and calculates that the extra income could fund a budget version of the trip to Patagonia I've spent the last few days dreaming about doing when this is all over. With little else on the menu, I may as well put myself through a month of twelve-hour days if that means something positive at the end.

Since I turned freelance a few years ago, things haven't always been easy. Finding a balance between having enough work to feed myself but not so much that there's barely time to do the feeding has been challenging. Only a year and a half ago, my full complement of clients shut down operations in the space of a single week. When I'd finally managed to rebuild a list of semi-reliable employers, the manic episode that landed me in hospital left me without them, too. The lesson learned was that saying 'no' to anything wasn't a luxury at my disposal, even when weeks of sleeplessness and stress had left my brain operating at a fraction of normal capacity.

I close the blinds and put in fourteen hours at my laptop, with a half-hour break to call Ma, Cath and Aiyla.

Later, somewhere into my second pack of the post-dinner biscuits I've been mindlessly shoving into my mouth for the last half-hour or so, I look up from the movie I'm watching on my laptop and see the pinking night sky through the window. I drop a half-eaten biscuit back onto the tray and go into the garden.

I sit on the lower tier of grass just as the last blush of daylight slips over the highest peak of the Orobie. The soft light speaks of a summer that's just around the corner. At this hour, the valley becomes a marmalade world in which everything is dimly golden, soft. Everything seems to move more slowly, sounds are muffled, and every angle is rounded and smoothed. My eyes burn from the lack of sleep and day at my computer, and my brain is thick with a fog I know won't lift until morning. I want to sit longer, much longer, but know if I do it will be harder to haul my body back up the steps and into bed when the fatigue that's already weighing down my limbs and eyelids has ripened.

As I traipse up the hill towards the door, with the town, mountains and emerging stars at my back, I have a feeling of having betrayed something. I feel a need to apologise, but to whom I am unsure.

Lockdown Day 28

Four weeks in quarantine.

Italy seems confused. The government in Lombardy has now made it compulsory to wear a mask when leaving home, two weeks after advising not to wear one unless infected. Over 100,000 people have been fined for breaching quarantine – 257 of them face fifteen years in prison for doing so after having tested positive for the virus, seven of them for driving to another *comune* in search of yeast. Mayors post videos of themselves removing the European flag from flagpoles and the press decries the rest of Europe's refusal to provide assistance, sparking an outcry among those who've been awaiting the discovery of just such a scapegoat for their frustrations. In the meantime, Austria,

Ukraine, Russia, Albania, Poland and Norway join China and Cuba in sending doctors by the dozen to help ease the strain on Italy's exhausted health system, and the Germans' ferrying of sick Italians into Saxony last week is forgotten.

America appears to be reaching the peak not of its coronavirus outbreak, but of the utter batshit-craziness it's been perfecting since 46.1 per cent of its voters gave batshit-craziness the rubber stamp circa four years ago. The news coming out of New York, in particular, is the stuff of nightmares – like a larger-scale version of what was happening in Bergamo a month ago. Of the 1,480 who died in the US yesterday, almost half were in New York. I've spent more than twelve months there in the past few years and in that time met around half the people I'd now call my closest friends in the world. We met at a climbing gym in Gowanus and climbed together daily after work in a group of five or six. On weekends we'd gather at 5 a.m. at a 24-hour bakery in Sunset Park, cram into a car and head north to climb on the Shawangunk Ridge until dark. All those friends are spread around Manhattan and Brooklyn, all of them in tiny apartments without gardens, without walls to climb, and without Giuseppinas.

I take my morning coffee to the terrace and sit in the strobes of morning sun threading the branches of the Japanese maple. A light dusting of snow fell on the higher peaks on Tuesday night but already I can see much of the snowpack has melted. It's hard not to think of where I'd be right now if none of this had happened.

I hear the baying of my neighbour Attilio's goats and stroll across the lawn to see whether they're still shut up in the stall on the far side of their garden or available for cuddles.

Before I've even reached the fence, I see the first of them bounding over towards me. He throws his front legs on top of the fence and dips his head for me to pet him. His tail is wagging and I realise I'm smiling – something I've done so little of in the past few weeks that it feels as though my lips have to break through the stiffness in my cheeks. I grab him a few handfuls of grass and let him eat from my hand, his coarse tongue tickling my skin.

'*Guarda giù là,*' a voice calls from somewhere obstructed by the wood pile stacked against the fence.

I shamble down the slope in my slippers and see Attilio squatting over a small shrub in his copse of fruit trees. He points to the bottom of the garden, where a second goat, the female, is trying to eat the leaves of a pear tree through a ring of protective fencing.

'Born on Monday,' Attilio shouts. 'Her name is Teresina.'

It's a few seconds before I spot what he's talking about.

Teresina is a tiny splotch of pristine white on the copper grass, so small that she might be an oversized snowball. She seems to be sleeping, until Attilio wolf-whistles. On cue, she jumps to her feet and performs a madcap trio of pirouettes before leaping towards her mother.

I am smitten.

'You can come over and pet her any time you want. Just make sure her momma is tied up ... She's very protective. And feisty!'

Ma calls while I'm in the garden attempting to cut the lawn with a short scythe taped to the end of a ski pole. Teresa and Teresina watch from the fence, nonplussed.

Ma gives me an update on the family. My cousin who

caught the virus has recovered. My dad's taking every chance he can get to escape to the beach and has amassed the materials – from Amazon and a hardware store in a nearby town – for at least a half-dozen DIY projects, but has started none. Two of my uncles have been furrowed.

'Fur*loughed*.'

'That's what I said, didn't I?' she says. 'Anyway, it's a silly word. Your aunt Helen got it too – fur*lough*ed. And I haven't heard much from Aunt Vic but she does that reiki business, so I don't suppose she'll be getting much in the way of work either. Oh, I'm so glad I'm retired, though I wouldn't mind a trip out of the—'

'Ma, sorry ... I have to go. I have a ton of work to get through and you always have to give me the director's cut of the family news.'

'Oh, I'm sorry. I just thought you might want to hear how everyone's doing and to wish me happy birthday.'

I glance at my watch and discover she's not mistaken. It is her birthday. Shit.

'Shit!' I say. 'I'm sorry, Ma! I've been so caught up in everything, I barely know what month we're in. Happy birthday!'

'Don't worry. As long as I know you and your sister are safe, that's the only present I need.'

I work in my bedroom, sunning my back at the window. The day is too perfect to venture outside and risk combusting with frustration.

In the mid-afternoon, I hear the voices of Enzo and his older daughter, Elisa. They're sunbathing in the garden.

'Did you hear about the ski-mountaineer on Monte Bianco?' Enzo asks me when I pull my chair down to join them. It must be well over 20 degrees but he's dressed in jeans, a thick sweater and a scarf.

'No, what happened?'

'Dead. Twenty-four years old. He broke quarantine and left on Saturday morning. They found him on Sunday below the Savoia hut. Silly bastard.'

'Poor thing,' says Elisa. 'He was my age.'

'Old enough to know better. Wouldn't you say, Kieran?'

'Nah. If it's in your blood, it's in your blood. It's a drug. The only surprise is that it hasn't happened more. Shit, if I didn't have all this work to do I'm sure I'd be giving it some consideration myself.'

'You're not serious, are you?' He takes off his sunglasses and tucks them over the collar of his sweater.

'Dad! You were going jogging every day yourself until the middle of March!'

'I'm not totally serious,' I say, 'but I can sympathise. If you'd asked me three months ago if I could go two or three months without climbing, without the mountains, I would have laughed. Supposing there are people out there who're more addicted than me, it makes sense that it happened – statistically, that is.'

'I've skied all my life. I haven't once thought about driving to Bormio and heading up Cima Bianca, or even up Sasso Nero in Valmalenco.'

'Really?' Elisa asks. 'Not even thought about it?'

'Okay, I may have thought about it,' Enzo says, 'but thinking and doing are different things. And when one puts other people's lives at risk and the other doesn't, the difference is big.'

'Dad, stop,' says Elisa, but he's already stopped. He's turned his head from her and is gazing over the valley towards Pizzo Meriggio, but from my angle I can see he isn't looking at anything. The sunlight catches something on his face and I see a tear drop from his chin onto his collar.

'I'm sorry,' he says, without turning back to face us. 'I'm just very tense.'

Elisa throws her sweater against his back.

'Papi, it's okay . . .' she says. Then, she leans towards me and whispers, 'Another of his colleagues died yesterday.'

We both sit there, two metres away, impotent.

Later that night, after climbing, I'm sitting at the window, finishing off my work for the day, when I hear music from one of the side streets around Via Scarpatetti. I roll up the blinds and look out over the town: the slate rooftops glisten like the scales of a fish, the head of the clock tower blushes in a thin stream of sun splitting the valley floor from west to east, the mountains look like ghosts of themselves in the purpling light. The subalpine strata of the mountainsides are turning green again. Wind hums through the vines and through the magnolia and walnut trees. To my right, the tricolore bats at half-mast on the battlement of Castel Masegra. If I could take only a handful of images to wherever it is I'll go when I die, this would be one of them. It is now a part of me.

In a lull in the music, I hear someone shouting somewhere between the castle and Fausto's plot at the top of Via Scarpatetti. A few seconds later, the music resumes, much louder than before. Instantly I recognise the haunting opening sequence of Andrea Bocelli's 'Con Te Partirò'. I feel a sudden hollowness in my stomach. My skin seems to pulse. Before even the first chorus, tears are flowing down my cheeks, but I can't close my eyes or look away.

The aria seems to float above the rooftops to the most distant peaks, gliding like a consoling hand along the length of the valley.

Lockdown Day 29

I have a situation within the situation. I've been trying to ignore it for a few days but today it's unavoidable. I haven't slept in days. I have all the symptoms – insomnia, anxiety, excessive emotionality, racing thoughts. I go to the bathroom cabinet and find I have nine pills left. I do the maths: if I go back to taking one a day, I'll have enough to see me through only to 15 April – two days past the official end of quarantine but fifteen short of the anticipated extension. Even if I go back to half a pill a day, my supply will run out on the 24th. Today I'm sure I need a whole pill, meaning I'll have even less time before my supply runs out.

I meet Giuseppina for our morning coffee at nine. She looks tired, but flashes me a sleepy grin as she takes her seat and looks down at me through the railing.

The coffee seems to refocus her eyes, and after we've been sitting for a few minutes I feel her watching me.

'What's troubling you?' she asks.

'A little insomnia,' I say. 'Nothing serious.'

'You're not alone. The days and nights are all much the same if you're in the one place all the time. Tonight I'll make you a dinner of pasta and beef, then you'll have a good sleep.'

A few seconds pass before she clicks.

'Ah, of course. Silly old woman! I sometimes forget that all this is happening. Well, get yourself a camomile tea and take some of the lavender from the garden and put it under your bed. That'll help.'

I stagger through the day. After four hours of work, I attempt a nap. I lie in bed, trying to convince myself I'm tired even though my body feels electrified, tense, wired. While I'm lying there, the mouse appears from some nook behind my wardrobe. He skirts gingerly along the base of my bookcase, pauses, then makes a dash across the no man's land of floor towards the door.

I follow him into the kitchen and go back to work.

I head to the wall at 6 p.m. to put in my quota of climbs. The neighbours are playing music again, this time opera I don't recognise, which is probably just as well. Each time the Bocelli song has appeared in my head throughout the day I've welled up, and it's doing nothing for my resilience. The chances of that happening again soon expire when the opera number ends and the unseen DJ selects 'Macarena' as his next track.

I call Aiyla when I'm done climbing.

'It's starting to sink in how long it will be before we see each other again,' she says. She's been doing online consultations and is dressed in her work outfit. The change is striking after a week of seeing her in pyjamas and gym clothes, but also a blessing of sorts, given the sexual urges that have manifested among the many side effects of quarantine but which no authority on such matters, as yet, has seen fit to include in their advisories on coping. 'Even three months from now, if you come here or I go to you, then we'll have to be in quarantine for, what, two weeks before we can see each other? And even then, will we be able to touch each other? I keep pretending you're away on military service, like all the teenage girls here. But I'm not a teenage girl, even if my family still treat me that way.'

The logistics in Turkey have always been tricky. Sneaking in phone calls and visits; only spending the odd night together, even then. Being unable to touch each other and hold hands in public in case a friend of the family should see. Now, things are only going to be all the more difficult.

'So, what are you saying?'

'It's shit! That's what I'm saying.'

'Ah, yeah. The shitness. Well, that goes without saying, really, doesn't it?'

'I just want it to all be over. To go back to normal.'

'Now you're behaving like a teenage girl.'

'I know!'

'Anyway, would you really want things to go back to exactly how they were?'

'Well, yeah. Don't you?'

'Not really. This whole thing has made me realise some things. Big things. Game-changers. And I think we're all learning lessons that we can't fathom just yet. I don't want to go back to taking everything for granted and feeling like I don't have enough time to sit in the garden at the end of the day and watch the sunset, or to call my mother. Or that I have to compensate myself for the drudgery of every day's work with a nightly Netflix-and-pretzel binge. I've slowed down – everyone has – and it's been eye-opening. It would have been blissful if it wasn't for the context. I think the value of things has increased, too, things that—'

Aiyla's face stiffens. Her hand flaps in front of the phone, blocking the camera. I hear her speaking to someone in the room and when she removes her hand she's not alone. Her mother is standing beside her, waving to me.

'*Merhaba*, Kieran,' she says.

'*Merhaba!*'

'It is very nice to finally meet you.'

She gives Aiyla a playful slap on the shoulder then disappears out of shot. I hear Aiyla's door closing behind her.

Aiyla turns back to the screen and drops her head into her hands.

'She knows!'

Aiyla is not religious, but her family are conservative, to the point of insisting she carries on living in the family home until she's married – nothing out of the ordinary for a 32-year-old in her world but far from conducive to uncomplicated courtship. Regular dating is, alas, out of the question. Having a boyfriend is out of the question. Having a Scottish, non-Muslim boyfriend is something we haven't dared broach.

'She's your mother,' I say. 'Of course she knows. She's probably known for a long time. Anyway, that didn't go too badly. It didn't seem like she was too upset that you were talking to me. Now you just have to tell your dad . . .'

Lockdown Day 30

Four hours' sleep. Not great, but better than no hours' sleep.

My doorbell rings at around 8 a.m. I spill my coffee over my t-shirt and pyjama trousers and gaze accusingly at the door.

It rings again. I put on my dressing gown and slippers, and shuffle across the room, opening the door carefully, like the idiot in the horror movies who shouldn't be opening the door. From the terrace, I look up to the front gate and see a human standing there in a mask and plastic visor, package in one hand and tablet in the other.

'Delivery for . . . eh . . .' He squints at the tablet.

'Cunningham?'

'That's the one.'

'We're still getting deliveries?'

'*Si, si.* We're behind with everything, but we're still running – on a limited schedule, of course. This one came from the UK. I'm surprised it made it.'

He hands me the parcel. I instantly recognise Ma's handwriting.

'Thank you very much.'

'You're welcome,' he says. 'Oh, we clean everything but I'd give it another wipe down before opening it. You never know ...'

I take the parcel into the kitchen, snip off the end, slide out its contents, deposit the packaging in the bin, then wash my hands and scissors and go back to the door to wipe down the handle.

I place the bundle of tissue paper and whatever's inside it – a book, it seems – on the kitchen table, then tear it open.

It's a Bible. A fucking Bible. Before I can call Ma and ask why she might have thought to put herself and Dad and me and every postal employee between us at risk by sending her Buddhist son a bloody Bible, I flip open the cover and find a Post-it with a smiley face and three kisses stuck to the first page. I pull it off. Below, a tiny jewellery box is nestled in a squarish cavity cut out of the centre of the pages.

I call Ma.

'Ma, it's arrived.'

'Your gran's ring?'

'Yeah.'

'Oh, I'm so happy. I thought we'd lost it!'

'Me too ... Well, I haven't really been able to think about it much the last little while, to be honest. Thank you, Ma. But what's with the Bible?'

'Well, we had to hide it somehow, in case someone pinched it. Your dad did it. I thought it was very clever. It's not blasphemous, is it?'

'I think it might be.'

'Anyway, don't you worry. All this will be over soon, then you can ask her.'

The plan had been hatched for Aiyla's next visit, which was scheduled for early June. She was going to teach for five days at a university in Ireland and had planned to stop off here on the way back, telling her family that she was sticking around in Ireland a few more days to see the sights.

'It won't be soon, Ma. Anyway, I only asked you to send it because I'd like to have it over here. Then, if the time comes and everything's still going well and she doesn't hate me already, I can—'

I realise mid-sentence what I should have realised a full ten minutes ago. I'd thought our mail had been blocked – at least the stuff from overseas.

'What's wrong?' Ma asks.

'When did you send this?'

'Well, I don't know. You asked me while you were still in Istanbul, I suppose. Then it took your dad a few days to get everything together and chop the middle out of all those pages, so probably about four weeks ago.'

Four weeks.

'Are you still getting mail?'

'Yes. We got a pair of clippers to cut the dog's hair today.

And something from Amazon. And your dad's been ordering all his things for the garden, too.'

'Ma, you've got to stop ordering stuff. Anything that comes through that door is your enemy. But, if you can, could you send something to me?'

'Of course, what do you want?'

When I get off the phone I shoot an email to the specialist's surgery in Edinburgh, explaining the situation. The secretary replies half an hour later telling me the meds will be in the mail by the end of the week, but can only be posted to the registered address. I make a transfer to the surgery account and call Ma back to tell her the meds will be arriving soon.

'Just be sure to wipe down the parcel when it comes and wash your hands after. When the mobile post office comes, wait until there's no queue, give him a tenner and tell him to keep the change. I'll pay you back in wine next time I'm home.'

I finish work at six, put in an hour on the Scorpion Wall, then sit on a thicket of weeds at the foot of the wall to watch another day ending.

While I'm sitting there and planning the night ahead – a quick dinner and early to bed – I get a sticky feeling, some mental itch I can't quite land a paw on to scratch. Something's making me uneasy. It takes me a while to get it, but when I do, the itch becomes a punch.

'I thought you were gonna go early to bed,' Aiyla says.

'So did I,' I say, 'but then I realised something.'

'What?'

'Well, everything I've been doing these past few weeks has been against everything I've ever believed in.'

'What, staying at home? You don't have much choice . . .'

'Nah, not that. I mean the killing time, shutting things out, turning my back on experience. I've been working fourteen-hour days, glued to my phone when I'm not on my laptop, closing the blinds, stuffing my face every night just to distract myself from my loneliness, sadness, anxiety, worry and all the other shit that's been dumped on us since this all began.'

'Everyone's doing that, honey,' she says. 'I think it's kinda normal. You're being too hard on yourself. I think you've been doing really well.'

'Only because I've been avoiding feeling anything.'

'I guess it depends on your definition of "well". Most people are just happy to get through days, whether there's a pandemic or not. Like I say, it's normal. It's self-preservation.'

'I guess. But it doesn't feel like any way to live. It just doesn't feel . . . human. I mean to only turn up for the good times. To say one kind of experience is worth my attention but another kind isn't.'

'What else could you do? I mean, would you like to be out there, helping in the hospitals or something like that?'

'No, it's not physical. It's mental and emotional. I should be braver; be present instead of distracting myself and hiding away in the world inside my computer screen or my phone; allow myself to experience things fully. I don't feel like shit because of the way things are, I feel like shit because I want them to be different. It just feels like a waste of life. And then there's Giuseppina. She needs me. All the years I've been here, I've always told myself she has her family so I don't need to be there for her like I would my own granny, but she's been lonely as hell since Domenico died and I've sat here, in my apartment, not 10 feet away from her through days when she hasn't seen anyone.

And she's lovely. Lovelier than ever. And wise. And funny. And smart as hell. How could I not have seen that before?'

'Do I need to be worried about this Giuseppina?'

'Don't joke.'

'I'm sorry. I was just trying to lighten the mood a little. Are you okay?'

I realise I've been raising my voice. I glance at the balconies on the buildings to my right for anyone who might've overheard, but it's dinner time and there's no one to be seen.

'Yeah, I'm fine,' I say. It's the first lie I've ever told her, but a quick conscience-check assures me it's a white one, for now. 'You don't have to be sorry. I'm just discovering that one of the reasons people don't like spending time with themselves is because they discover their selves aren't as likeable or impressive or decent as they can allow themselves to think when they're with others. I'm a case in point.'

'Go to bed,' she says. 'I can see you're tired and that's not helping you at all. You do what you can, and the fact that Giuseppina treats you like one of her own, despite all that you say, should tell you it's all in your head. If you decide to spend more time with her in future, cut down on work and try to open up to whatever's going on inside you, great, but don't beat yourself up about what you've done to get by in the past.'

Before bed, I write an email to my client asking to reduce my workload for the month. Patagonia can wait, but Italy can't.

Lockdown Day 31

I work from 2 a.m. to 8 a.m. then take a break to climb, hoping it will help me have a nap later. I've been doing recce on two other walls with potential for climbing and want to give them a try.

The first is the retaining wall between the top of the vineyard and the patch of lawn at the front of the house – a crumbling, six- or seven-metre stretch of rounded stones set in decaying concrete. The second is on the west-facing wall of the house, directly below both of our kitchens. If I can establish doable routes on both, I'll have enough variety to keep myself busy and entertained even if lockdown is extended to the end of May.

I play around on the new walls for two hours. Neither is likely to become a classic, but they're good enough to provide a little more motivation.

A Guide to the Walls of No. 3
Via Aurelio Fracassetti

The Scorpion Wall

Length: 5 metres (8 with extension to corner of eastern wall)

Difficulty: 5a* (6a with two fingers; 6a+ gastons† only; 6b+ one hand only)

Notable features: Bird's nest on upper western portion of wall,

---

* Italy uses the French grading system for sport-climbing routes. The system ascends from 1 (walking) through 9c, which is the hardest climb completed to date. Numerical grades are given by the first person to climb the route and are subdivided by adding a letter (a, b or c) and a '+'. The mean grade of regular climbers is roughly 6a.

† A technique that involves pushing outward on holds as opposed to pulling down or towards the body.

beneath balcony; bedroom windowsill; fist-jam pocket just past the bedroom dihedral has a scorpion inside.

Comments: A pleasurable, vertical granite pitch with alternating juggy* and crimpy† handholds and plentiful slots for foot placements, though these are occasionally dusty and become slick after rain.

The Dusk Wall

Length: 20 metres approx.

Difficulty: 5c

Notable features: Large steel pole protruding at head height after 4.5 metres (duck); slippery little bastard of a foot placement on serpentine block before final move prior to reaching Benedetta's granny's gable wall.

Comments: A delightful long traverse on a south-facing wall composed of blocks of granite, schist, serpentine and a lump or two of gneiss. Outstanding views and crimpy holds. Occasional loose rocks add a further element of 'interest' and a surprising crux appears mid-route when the large toe pockets turn to pocks for a stretch of 3–4 metres.

The Dirty Wall

Length: 7 metres

Difficulty: 5b (5c after rain)

Notable features: Bail-out option above, courtesy of railing around

---

* Large, jug-like cavities or protrusions that can be grasped easily.
† Small; for fingertips only.

lower patch of lawn; extensive ivy on western and eastern portions; flaky cement.

Comments: This largely unfrequented crag features a 6–7-metre traverse over footholds of invariably loose rock with rotting concrete for the hands and occasional patches of moss.

Indecent Exposure

Length: 6 metres

Difficulty: 6a+

Notable features: Giuseppina's rose bush; cellar door; kitchen window and sill; pipe.

Comments: An airy, exposed and physical pitch that involves a dynamic swinging manoeuvre over the cellar door and then stemming around the corner to the kitchen window via a slightly loose water pipe.

I call Ma when I'm done climbing.

'Your dad's been a little bit nervous,' she whispers. 'He doesn't do well with all this being cooped up, and when he goes out he gets anxious about people coming too close to him.'

I hear their doorbell ring. The dog goes apeshit, though not apeshit enough that I can't hear Pa growl a swear word in the background.

'*Oh no!*' says Ma. 'I'll be right back.'

'Ma, go to the window – don't go to the do—'

She's gone, but has left the phone on.

'I'll be right the-ere,' Ma calls in her visitor voice.

'Tell whoever it is to bugger off,' Pa says. '*Tits!*'

'Shhh . . . It's Lizzy and her pal Mark, the chap from the chemist's!'

'I couldn't give a toss if it's ...'

Lizzy is Ma's recently divorced friend from the village. About two days prior to lockdown in the UK, she appointed Ma her designated bestie and shoulder to cry on. I sympathise, but not enough that I want her anywhere near my slightly aged, high-risk and highly strung parents.

I hear Ma explaining the no-visitors policy, one Lizzy's already heard several times before, I imagine.

A few minutes pass before Ma says goodbye and closes the door.

I hear her tromping back along the hallway.

'For goodness sake!' she says.

'Next time,' Pa says, 'I'll answer.'

It's at least five minutes before she returns to the phone.

'Sorry, son,' she says. 'It was Lizzy and Mark. They brought me flowers and I had to put them in the bin and then wash my hands and disinfect the doorbell. They're away along the street together now, barely even a foot apart.'

'You need to be harder with them. They're not getting it. Let Dad answer next time, like he says.'

'I'll do no such thing. I don't know what he'd say.'

'Probably what you should've been saying to them since they started coming two weeks ago.'

'No, I'll phone her tonight. I'll just say we're very uptight and won't be answering the door in future. That's alright, isn't it?'

'Mum,' I say – I only ever call my mum 'Mum' when it's serious – 'You're in the middle of a life-threatening pandemic. Anything is alright. Waving a pitchfork would be almost mannerly. Going around ringing people's doorbells pretty much excuses any kind of response short of shooting them.'

The call to Ma puts me more on edge than anything else I've experienced these past weeks. I pull open my kitchen drawer to look for a cigarette, then remember I don't smoke any more.

The nap isn't going to happen. I grab my meditation cushion and take it to the garden to sit beneath the magnolia tree.

I sit for two hours, put in four hours of work in the afternoon, then return to the Dusk Wall for my evening session.

Lockdown Day 33

Good Friday.

People aren't singing on their balconies any more. The kids are no longer making the *'Andrà tutto bene'* (Everything will be okay) posters displayed in windows and on balconies a month ago. Giuseppe Conte, the Italian prime minister, looks ready to collapse. Everyone knows now that it won't be *tutto bene*, that we're already past that and the fallout is going to be huge. And long. And hard. The US president tweeted last night that the economy will bounce back quickly. The International Monetary Fund says we're in for the worst recession since the Depression. I know little of these things, but know which I'm inclined to trust.

I can't shake the feeling that this pandemic is only beginning, not ending; that the concentrated, intensive war that's been waged against it thus far is about to descend into one of attrition, with no end in sight.

I wake at 2 a.m., feeling like I've had ten cups of coffee. On my way to the bathroom, I glance back into the living room and see Pa sitting in the Lazy Boy chair by the window, drinking a cup of tea while poring over a map of the route we have planned for later in the day. He's real for a full second before I realise I'm dreaming.

Mid-pee, I catch a glimpse of myself in the mirror. My hair's wild, my eyes wilder still. I instinctively look down at my hand for the other tell that I've come to rely on these past few years. It's shaking. I take my meds from the drawer beneath the sink and swallow another one. Five left.

I try to do my work for the day before dawn, hoping I'll be able to rest later, but it doesn't happen. I scan the news instead. I discover that Lombardy's lockdown will be extended to 3 May. It's not the best start.

Later, I meet Giuseppina for morning coffee outside. Today she isn't wearing her jacket or bathrobe: summer is coming.

'Another day,' she says, with more enthusiasm than seems feasible, until I recall the date and remember that today the family will visit.

'Another day,' I repeat, trying my best to muster a smile.

The sun has already climbed above the horizon and is threatening further splendour. I look behind me and see that the peak of Punto di Santo Stefano is already piebald, having shed at least half of its winter cloak.

Ma calls a little after lunchtime. I've abandoned work and am in the garden with the ski-pole scythe, swatting at dandelions and daisies that have undergone an overnight resurrection worthy of Jesus himself.

'They arrived!' she says, sans introduction.

'Who arrived?'

'Your pills. The postal van won't be coming until Monday morning, but I'll pop around then and they'll be on their way. With any luck, they'll be with you by Friday. And don't worry, I'll—'

'Ma, stop . . .'

A pang of guilt slaps me out of the torpor with which the afternoon sun and sleeplessness have addled my brain. In the past few days, the daily death toll in the UK has pipped the thousand mark and infection rates have skyrocketed.

'What is it?'

I can forgive myself a lie far more easily than I could responsibility for infecting my high-risk, asthma-suffering mother. And I'd rather run the risk of an episode than spend five to fourteen days waiting for the moment when she calls showing symptoms.

'Ma, I'm sorry. I totally forgot. I found another pack under the bathroom sink the other day. I was going to call and tell you but I must have got distracted.'

'Are you sure there's enough to keep you going?'

'I'm sure, Ma.'

'And you will be able to speak to someone who can help if you need them, won't you?'

'Yes. Stop worrying.'

'It's just we know it hasn't always been easy over there, that they maybe don't have quite the same sympathy and under-standing of these things as in other places. It's not a criticism; I just always remember the problems you've had in the past.'

The stigma and hush-hushery surrounding mental health issues in Italy is as strong and diffuse as anywhere I've ever been. It is, to date, the only downside I've discovered to living here.

Shortly after arriving in Italy, I made the decision to be more open about my experience with Bipolar, both out of a sense of obligation to do whatever I could to reduce stigma and raise awareness, and a growing appreciation of how critical communication is as a coping mechanism.

Before coming here, I'd always felt set apart. I'd been a recluse, not because of any misanthropic convictions but because, until then, each of my attempts to find my place in the world had ended in disappointment and done little more than convince me of my otherness. Here, I'd come to feel a sense of belonging and acceptance I'd never known before. I had friends, a job I didn't hate, students I adored and a cleaner bill of health than I'd enjoyed anywhere. While the topography helped, I'd learned for once to feel as comfortable among people and as I did alone and at altitude. For the first time in my life, I'd seen scope for flourishing instead of merely surviving. This, however, was dependent on forming lasting and meaningful relationships, something that couldn't be done – not really – while my non-disclosure of pertinent particulars kept anyone I might form them with at arm's length.

But 'coming out' hasn't always been easy. Each time, the stress entailed in building up the courage to spill the beans to a potentially unsympathetic listener has triggered small bouts of anxiety and insomnia, and some of the reactions I've encountered along the way have tested my resolve to make forthcomingness a matter of policy. An ex-boss wondered, audibly, if my condition was 'what Rain Man had'. A few climbing partners swiftly became other people's climbing partners. One friend pumped his eyebrows a few times, as though I'd confessed the nought-to-sixty capabilities of my car, not the biochemical misfortunes of my brain, then made no further mention of the confession for as long as I knew him. A girl I was dating told me she'd once seen a documentary about schizophrenia ('Or was it split-personality disorder?') and asked if I could be, in any way, 'y'know – dangerous'. Others responded more kindly but warned against sharing the disclosure liberally.

When I bemoaned the above to a therapist I visited a few years ago, she reminded me I was lucky not to live in the days of Mussolini and Hitler, when those diagnosed with mental illness were tossed into foibas, mineshafts or gas chambers along with Jews and objectors.

Each time I encountered such reactions, the clocks seemed to have been rewound, the true way of things restored, and I felt as though I'd been deposited into a world no different to the bleak, inhospitable place I'd wandered out into when first diagnosed; one that didn't particularly want me in it, that would tolerate me only inasmuch as I could maintain a ruse of being other than what I was, of being 'normal'. Maybe, I thought, Sondrio wouldn't be the perfect, forever home I'd envisioned.

It wasn't until I met Lucia, Gaia, Simona, Giulia, Luigi, Matteo, David, and the rest of those who are now my closest friends in the valley, that I finally understood – just as the illness itself has varying degrees of severity, the human capacity for empathy, compassion, and understanding has its own spectrum. And while there are places where prevailing attitudes have evolved to a greater or lesser extent than elsewhere, within each there are plenty of benignant parts that temper the benightedness of the whole. It's just a matter of finding them, something more likely done with the news out there than otherwise. The therapist was right, in a way, but just as. we might now be appalled by how sufferers of mental illnesses were treated a century ago, getting to the stage where we might one day look back and be appalled at the stigma that still exists today requires honesty, openness, bravery and unwavering commitment to talking as freely about our headstuff as we do the rest of it, irrespective of the anticipated response.

Even, maybe, in the middle of a pandemic.

I go back to work in the garden, putting in a few hours with the shears to quash the worst of the weeds and unruly grass around the borders on the west side of the house. I'm on the narrow strip of grass below Giuseppina's kitchen, alternately trimming and yanking out rat's-tail, horsetail and nightshade around the stone surround of the flowerbed against the wall, when I catch the scent of cigarette smoke. The smell is delicious and, somehow, heartening – weak enough that I know the smoker isn't near, but strong enough that it allows me to feel momentarily blessed with a crumb of companionship.

Lockdown Day 34

I call Aiyla in the morning. Late yesterday afternoon, the Turkish government announced a 48-hour quarantine running from midnight on Friday to midnight on Sunday.

'They gave us no warning!' she tells me. 'I'm glad they have finally done something but last night the city was chaos. People were fighting in the streets to get inside the markets and bakeries.'

I hear a chicken in the background.

'You have chickens in Istanbul?'

'I know, right? It's so silent!'

Her look turns pensive.

'Today you seem . . . I forgot the word.' She plucks the mini dictionary she keeps on her desk and flicks through the pages.

'*Woebegone*. Is that right?'

'Glum?'

'Yeah, *glum*.'

'I just keep thinking about what the consequences are going to be.'

'Herd immunity, probably.'

'No,' I say, guessing something's been lost in translation, like the day she told me she had an 'inbred' toenail. 'That's a sort of strategy that says once we've all had it, then we'll have a collective resistance to infection because so many will have developed antibodies.'

'Thanks for the mansplain, Doctor Cunningham, but I don't mean to the virus. I mean crowd immunity to lies and death and shitting on people's personal liberties and all that. All these things are becoming normalised, and the longer we're exposed to them, the greater the tolerance we develop for them. For example, everyone here knows the death toll is much higher than is being reported, but our leaders continue to cook the numbers so people believe they're competent and don't have to shut down the economy. And that idiot in the US – he's the most powerful man in the world and he's saying one thing one second then denying he said it ten seconds later. And people are already accepting that. Lying's been rubber-stamped. Then there's the injustice – all the Black people and Hispanics dying in America, the nurses getting screwed over in the UK, then all these rich white people in

Europe and the US moaning about how hard they have it when we all know that this is only foreplay, that the true fucking's going to come if this really takes off in India, Africa, Syria, South America. We should be rioting – instead, we're sitting on our couches, distracting ourselves with comfort food and Netflix.'

I make another coffee and head outside to see if Giuseppina's there to join me. I call Ma while I'm waiting for her to appear.

'Now, don't worry,' she says, her voice like a shaken bag of coal. 'Your dad and I have a wee bit of a cough and sore throats, and he says he has some aches and pains, but we're fine. We've been taking our temperatures every few hours and they're perfectly normal. I just thought it best to tell you rather than leave you guessing.'

My gut tied itself into a knot after her first three words. My chest feels like it's harbouring a drummer banging his way through my solar plexus. This – *this* – is my worst nightmare. The unthinkable.

I call her or my dad every hour or two through the day.

I'm angry. Ma hasn't left the house in three weeks, but only two days ago Pa went for a walk with a friend. He takes the dog for walks daily on the beach or in the forest behind the village. He orders a new book or piece of DIY kit almost every day on Amazon. But how can you be angry with your father when you're scared he's infected with a potentially fatal disease?

Between calls home and to my sister, I climb, spending an hour on each wall. After my first traverse, I notice that the minor paunch I developed at the start of quarantine has gone, burned away by the nervous energy of the last few weeks. My ribs are visible and my tummy has sunk below my hip bones.

I feel surprisingly strong, though suspect my edginess has lent fuel to my body.

For the first hour, on the Dusk Wall, the darker rocks are almost too hot to touch. After every traverse I take out my phone to check for any updates from Ma, the first time being only ten minutes after we'd spoken. After my first call home, I head to the Scorpion Wall, determined to climb slowly and deliberately, to make it an exercise in mindfulness.

I start with my right hand cupped around a head-high block on the arête formed by the south- and east-facing walls. I place the toe of my right foot into a two-centimetre gap between two stones at my hip, crimp on a two-finger slit almost parallel to my right hand, and push up with my right foot. While the rest of the climb may be bordering on banal, in this short initial transition from grounded to airborne I feel the same energising, liberating rush I feel on any crag or cliff, like a departure from one world to another. I bring my right hand over below my left, hook my right toe around the arête, and drop my weight to reach with my left hand for a three-inch flake two feet to the side. After releasing my right toe from the arête, I press it into a tiny fissure above the left, push down, and spread my left onto the bevelled corner of a smaller block two feet to the left. Already my breathing is calmer, my body harmonised in a way it never can be on horizontal ground. I lay three fingers on the last block before the stucco panel below the bedroom window, placing them down gently to feel the coarse rub of the granite and shift to find the optimal spot for traction. I bring my feet together below me and undercling a slightly protruding block at waist height with the middle and ring fingers on my left hand. I step up with both feet onto the next block, pressing my weight into the wall until my cheek is against the stucco panelling, bring the right hand in beside my left, then throw the left out to a side-pull at full stretch. I bring my right hand into a vertical crack at my navel and squeeze inwards on both holds, using the tension to support my weight while I stretch to a pocket with my left foot and squeeze the toe of my right into a slit just above the left. I shift my weight onto my left foot, raise my right so the toe just touches the surface of the wall for balance, tuck two fingers on my right hand into a cementy crack at chest height, then reach for a high jug on the left. After matching hands on the jug, the difficulties are over. I switch feet below me, and at full wingspan can grab hold of a huge flake on the opposing arête and shake out one arm at a time before doing it all in reverse.

I call Ma and Pa one last time at around 9 p.m. They're in the living room, watching TV. They're still at a stable 36.5 degrees, but both are coughing, and both have flu-like aches throughout their bodies.

The news: South Korea is using tracking wristbands on those who defy quarantine orders. China has banned publication of academic research on the origin of the virus. The US death toll has overtaken Italy's. The number of confirmed cases worldwide is approaching 2 million. An eagle is spotted flying over central Milan.

My parents might have coronavirus.

Lockdown Day 35

Easter Sunday.

I wake in the night, but this time the awakening is welcome.

I can smell it before I hear it. Hear it before I see it. The *föhn*. Every year when this warm mountain wind arrives, it's like meeting an old friend. She comes bearing gifts: a concentrated miasma of scents from the alpine world above, made all the more enchanting by its current inaccessibility.

I walk onto the lawn in my bare feet, enjoying the cool grass and earth. Little bits of summer are stuck in the night air and rise out of the earth like *petites madeleines* of childhood. The night pulses, pregnant with unknown mischief. The moon, neatly aligned above the pointed tip of Pizzo di Rodes, looks like a giant shortbread round someone's taken a bite out of. An orgy of stars throbs either side of it, the world below spangled by their light.

The sun and moon traverse the sky. I traverse the walls, the bed, the days. And yet it moves.

I head to the Scorpion Wall before dawn and put in twenty traverses without stopping, then sit for meditation. The day is unmistakably summery, upward of 20 degrees. I can't remember such a sustained spell of perfect weather in all the time I've been here.

I call Ma as soon as I think is decent and find out she and Pa had a good night. They're still coughing but their temperatures are low and the aches are easing off.

'Maybe we overdid it with the yoga the day before,' she tells me.

Luca texts around 10 a.m., telling me he's in the garden with Giuseppina. I find them yelling at each other over the patch of lawn below the Scorpion Wall, with Giuseppina on the swinging chair below my living room window, Luca on the top of the retaining wall that forms the Dirty Wall. They're a full 10 feet apart.

'It's necessary,' says Luca. 'I took the week off work to volunteer at the hospital in Padova. They have a new system. I wasn't flying patients to the hospital but flying doctors to patients at accident sites: one lady who had a kitchen fire and first-degree burns all over her face; another who slipped in the shower; a man who was drilling into plasterboard without protective glasses and then hit brick ... Then, every night, at least one accident for the delivery people – they're the only ones on the streets, dozens of them on bikes and mopeds. Some fall off, some crash into each other, and one even slipped down two flights of stairs in an apartment block.'

'I remember Padova well,' says Giuseppina. 'Domenico took me to see all the old churches and *palazzi*. Such a beautiful city. I remember the markets and cafés around the edges of the squares. It very well may have been at Easter time, too. Back then, we always used to buy a new dress for Easter so we could go for picnics on *pasquetta* (Easter Monday). I don't suppose there will be any need this year.'

'You wouldn't like to see it now, *Nonna*,' says Luca. 'Here, there aren't so many people going around at the best of times, but there it's normally buzzing. Without any people it's a sad place.'

'Well, we'll have our own little Easter here all the same. Will you come this afternoon, Kieran? We're going to have the *colomba* in the garden.'

I meet them in the garden at 4 p.m. – Giuseppina, Enzo, Cristina, Monica, Elisa and Anna. Four of us sit on the grass on the lower tier and three on the upper tier. Monica, in gloves, mask, apron and hairnet, serves us each a slice of the cake and a glass of prosecco.

Enzo tells me his insurance business is already starting to take a hit.

'People don't have money to take out policies, so it looks like they're just going to do without. A lot of the policies – house insurance, life insurance, pet insurance – are seen as optional, so they're the first thing to go when things are tight.'

Cristina tells me that Luca couldn't make it because he's wiped out from his shifts in Padova. Her husband, who is head of the regional mountain rescue team, has taken a team to patrol the major trailheads and tourist areas with police to ensure no hikers try to take advantage of the good weather with a day in the mountains. She's spent the day speaking to an old university friend whose father died in a hospital near Bergamo two weeks ago. The friend, along with dozens of others whose family members have died, are suing the hospital for refusing them treatment because they were over sixty-five.

'Wait,' says Anna. 'That just doesn't make sense. If they sue the hospital, then the hospital has even less money to buy ventilators and all that, so they'll be forced to let more people die.'

'The argument is that they should have had enough in the first place. Only in Italy! Kieran, would anything like this ever happen in the UK? I doubt it . . .'

'You'd be surprised . . .'

'Enough!'

Giuseppina is slapping the rug they've placed for her in the middle of the lower tier.

'Enough of this talk about the dead and the hospitals and this virus. It's Easter!'

'She's right,' says Elisa. 'We talk about nothing but this shit all day, every day.'

'Mind your language!'

'Sorry, *Nonna*. But you know what I mean . . .'

We sit in awkward silence until I head back inside to text Ma. As I'm climbing the stairs, Monica says, 'Andrea Bocelli's doing a live concert at the Duomo tonight. It'll be on YouTube.'

I watch it later. The stream opens with aerial footage of Milan: the canals of Navigli, Sforzesco Castle, then the Duomo, the giant Gothic cathedral in the city centre. The organ starts up. Bocelli, dressed in a tux, appears in the apse and opens with 'Panis Angelicus'. Throughout the hymn, the footage switches between Bocelli and a montage of images from Bergamo, Brescia and elsewhere around Lombardy. This, somehow, more than any newspaper report or anything else on social media, drills home the scope of this thing, that it is happening beyond the limits of the horizon I see from my apartment windows.

By the end of 'Ave Maria', I'm on my second tissue. For his final song, 'Amazing Grace', Bocelli moves outside onto the steps in front of the Duomo in the giant Piazza, reminding me of a day I spent there with Ma about four years ago during *Carnavale*, when a queue ten deep and forty wide waited to get inside the cathedral and thousands of Milanese in costumes frolicked around the city. Before the song finishes I switch off, slap shut my laptop and trudge through to bed.

I've texted Ma throughout the day. Each time she's replied with the same: *'36.3 & 36.5 xxx.'* I call to discover she and Pa are neither better nor worse, tell her I love her, and, for the first time, suffer the first thought that I may never see her or Pa or home again. I mean, the scenario doesn't seem too implausible – one in which this thing continues indefinitely, peaking and troughing, with no vaccine or end in sight, and no way home. Alone in this apartment, there are few barriers to these leaps of thought. I know they're wild, but no wilder than assuming the world's going to continue as before on 4 May. No wilder, indeed, than all *this* would've seemed to us just a few months ago.

I return to the garden after dark and lie on the grass with my MP3 player and headphones. I've already added the Bocelli version of 'Ave Maria' to a playlist that includes 'Hymn of the Cherubim', Barber's 'Adagio for Strings', 'Flamenco Sketches' by Miles Davis and 'Pavane' by Gabriel Fauré. The playlist is marked X and the last time I listened to it was probably the night before the morning when Luca found me unconscious in the garden. I don't know if it's a trigger or an accompaniment, but every note of every song harmonises perfectly with my mood. Everything is so harrowingly beautiful it hurts; everything's so hurtful it's somehow beautiful.

I lie there, knowing I should be inside, trying to sleep, doing my breathing exercises, going through my five-point list of containment strategies, calling Ma or Pa or Cath or Aiyla to let them know what I'm still trying to kid myself I don't know. Anyway, it might not come to anything, right? And the feeling is magical, so magical that it's easy to overrule, to ignore the red flags. Part of me is aware; part of me curses the awareness. Part of me wants to shut down before it's too late, the other to give myself over unconditionally to the rapture.

Lockdown Day 36

Three hours' sleep.

Status report: blue, with occasional shades of lilac.

I call Ma while I'm doing my traverses on the Dusk Wall. She and Pa are doing better. Their temperatures haven't gone above 36.5 and their coughs are no worse than yesterday.

Aiyla tells me the Turkish minister of internal affairs resigned last night for his part in the grocery stampede on Friday night.

'This country is like a barn,' she tells me. 'It was already barn-like before all this, but now it's like there's a wolf in there making all the animals nuttier than ever.'

'How nutty are you? Scale of one to ten.'

'I'd say a solid seven, but my bonsai tree might disagree. It's feeling harassed by all the attention I've been giving it. What about you? Scale of one to ten.'

'You know I'm not sleeping.'

'Yeah, I know. Do you feel something coming?'

'Nah, I'm fine. Seriously. I'll sleep eventually. If something bad was coming you'd notice by now, I promise.'

'Unless you didn't want to worry me and were a very good actor.'

'I'm not.'

'You told me not to believe you when you're manic because you'll tell me you're not manic. So what do I do? Are you taking your medication?'

'Yep.'

'Promise?'

'Promise.'

Next, I text Holly.

'Holly, I think I need your help.'

'Hey. Shit. You okay?'

'Yeah . . .

'Nah . . .

'I don't know . . .

'I mean, I'm okay now, I think, but there's a chance I might not be soon.

'Running out of meds.

'Been taking a half-dose for the last few weeks.

'Probably should be taking a higher dose to deal with everything . . .'

'Say no more,' she texts back. *'Take a pic of your prescription or the medication box and I'll see what I can do.'*

I need to move. I still have enough food supplies for at least another week but after an hour on the walls I get dressed, mask up, throw on a backpack and head to the supermarket.

I deliberately choose the town's most distant supermarket and make it all the way without seeing anyone. I discover why when I reach the entrance, which is closed and has a sign posted on the front window that reminds me it's *pasquetta*. The round trip takes only half an hour, but when I reach home I feel reinvigorated, calmed and almost regret contacting Holly. At the top of Via Scarpatetti I see two old ladies whom I used to pass every day when I worked as a teacher. No matter the day or hour, they could be found going door to door in their wool (winter) or floral (summer) dresses, pinafores and leather shoes, doing rounds of their cronies sitting on terraces or balconies. Both of them wear slightly dazed expressions, as if they still haven't quite grasped what's happening.

'Buongiorno,' I say, trying to smile, then realise I'm wearing a mask.

'We were just saying,' says the taller of the two, the only one I've ever heard speak, 'we miss those days when you'd come sprinting down the hill on your way to work. It gave us a laugh every morning.'

I ask if I can help them with anything. They must be well into their nineties and I've never seen either with family members.

'We are well. As well as can be, anyway. We have our own community on this street. We help each other to get by, irrespective of what they're doing in the rest of Italy. And our gallivanting years are long past, so it's no great trouble being confined to the neighbourhood. But it must be wearying for you young folk ... The time drags, doesn't it?'

'A bit, yes.'

'Don't you worry, *ragazzo*. You've plenty to spare. You look after yourself,' she says. 'It's a terrible time to be all alone. If this virus wasn't going about, I'd tell you to come for a plate of pasta. You've been losing weight cooped up on your own.'

'*Sarà per la prossima volta,*' I tell her. Maybe next time.

A few steps up the street I stop.

'Sorry,' I say, turning around. 'I've never asked your names.'

'I'm Maria Grazia,' says the taller one, 'and this is Maria Rosa.'

'It's a pleasure to meet you both.'

'*Altretanto,*' she says, smiling as she nods, and turns back to greet the lady who's appeared on the stairs above.

Lockdown Day 37

When I wake, it's gone. The mania, that is.

I don't know how, but it's no longer there. I'm sure of it. I pull my hand out from under the covers and hold it in front of my face. There is no wobble, no shake. I've rapid-cycled before, but this is abrupt and lacking the usual long, kamikaze descent careening through ever-thickening clouds of anxiety, irritability and irrationality on my way to a crash landing.

Maybe a lull? I go to the bathroom and take half a pill. My body and brain feel sluggish, but not the kind of sluggish that would suggest an impending depressive rebound, at least not a heavy one. In a way the physical torpor is a welcome reprieve from the tension and wiredness brought on by these past few weeks' insomnia, but the substitute is a soporific haze and a feeling of insuperable heartbreak, like someone's taken something away from me that I can never have back, even if I don't know what that thing is.

The day's a wipeout. This happens. After manic spells, no matter how short-lived, there comes an inevitable spell of low energy, the depth and length of which usually corresponds with the intensity and length of the preceding high. At some point, I realise I still have deadlines to meet and now none of the nervous energy that will let me fire off my usual output, but I don't care. I shut the blinds and stay in bed most of the day, getting up only to go to the bathroom and refill the cups of coffee that do little to reanimate me.

I text Ma instead of calling.

'36.5?'

'Hi darling. Yes. 36.5 again. I still have the cough but it's easing up a bit. Watching a film on Netflicks in my jammies. Are you okay, pet?'

'I'm fine . . . Just busy with work.

'Don't worry if you don't hear from me later.

'Just let me know you are okay.'

'Okay darling xxx.'

At around 3 p.m. I hear Giuseppina on the stairs and then a knock on my door. I lie still until I hear her retreating footsteps – today, I know, my company would be more of a burden than a welcome break from the monotony.

I stay in bed until dinner time, when I'll be unlikely to see anyone, and return to the Dusk Wall to try a few traverses. I can't even make it a quarter of the way through the first traverse. My legs feel shot with lead, my arms limp, my brain foggy, eyes blind to the presence of holds. I step back and retreat to the start of the climb, but this time come up even shorter.

I slump against the foot of the wall to read the news, none of which alleviates my mood.

Before bed I try to leaven my mood with a film – one of the old *Fantozzi* movies, which are to Italian culture what *Monty Python* is to British. Before it's ten minutes in, I switch off, slap shut my laptop and shuffle through to my bed. My bed is no longer just the place I sleep but a portal into tomorrow, one step closer to this thing's end.

Lockdown Day 38

Giuseppina comes to the door again around noon. This time I force myself out of my bed and answer.

'Ciao!' she says. Her huge smile almost forces me into one of my own. 'I haven't seen you. I wanted to know you are okay.'

Behind her, another beautiful day is brewing.

'I'm fine. Just very tired. I've been working too much, I think.'

'I told you!'

'Yes, you did.'

I realise I haven't changed clothes in days, nor showered, and take a step back from the doorway.

'The girls can't come today. I was wondering if you'd like to join me outside for a coffee.'

'I should really go back to bed,' I tell her. 'I had a bit of a headache through the night.'

She puts her hands on her hips, knuckles closed in fists, and pouts her lips into a frown.

'Will I have to come in there and drag you outside? Put some slippers on. I'll make the coffee. I'm not my best today either. I'm hoping a little bit of sunlight and fresh air might help.'

Five minutes later she reappears and leaves a steaming cup of coffee at the top of the landing. After fetching it, I drag my chair to the lawn so I can see her.

'There, now,' she says. 'Just you sit there and let the fresh air in about you. The pair of us will soon be all the better for it. Have you spoken with your parents? They okay?'

'Yes, they're better, thank you. And thank you for the coffee.'

'So many thank-yous,' she says, waving a hand in the circular motion that, to Italians, indicates excess. 'When we start thanking each other for common decency, I think we're lost.'

I can't help but smile. If she could be bottled, she'd sell out quicker than yeast.

'Such beautiful days we are having,' she says. 'Can you ever remember a spring like it?'

I shake my head.

'You're missing your mountains, I imagine.'

'Yes. And my parents, and Aiyla, and my friends.'

'Yes, of course. But you mustn't be despondent. One day, trust me, you'll miss all of this too.'

The loss of vitality and strength during depressive swings is always surprising, no matter how many times it's happened before. There's always cognitive bias, I think, in our reckoning of our own capabilities, and the disconnect between what we'd like to believe and reality is only widened further for Bipolars by the stark discrepancy between our operating capacity when manic compared with when depressive. I'm particularly guilty of this, reading the inertia of my 'down' spells as the anomaly and perceiving the high energy and productiveness of my 'up' spells as the norm, as 'Me'.

I have no idea what to expect in the weeks ahead. The last time I cycled so quickly, the manic symptoms returned soon after the first dip, and there isn't a 'last time when I've been Bipolar in a pandemic'. I took my last half-pill this morning. Now, I find myself 'free-solo' in the biggest challenge of my life. I'd always expected to meet that challenge in the Himalayas, maybe Pakistan, maybe the wilds of Alaska or on one of the legendary monoliths of Yosemite. Instead, it's happening a little above sea level in a one-bed apartment in a small town in northern Italy.

Later, another knock on the door. I'd been expecting it.

'You aren't busy, are you?'

'No,' I say. 'I've just been trying to do some work, but it's not really happening.'

'In that case, I may have a job for you.'

She leads me up the stairs and along the back of the house to the shed.

'Cristina brought me this last week,' she says, pointing to an eight-foot palm leaning against the back of the shed. 'She had it outside her apartment but she says it's too big. It was blocking the light. I was thinking we could put it near the fence; that way we'll have a little more privacy from the neighbours and I won't have to see the mess they're making with that new wall of theirs.'

I haul the tree down to the lawn and dig a two-foot-deep hole in the second tier, a yard from the fence. It takes an hour to get the thing balanced and pack in enough soil to keep it upright. When done, I realise I haven't had a single thought about the virus.

Lockdown Day 41

I call Ma in the morning.

'I had an awful night,' she tells me. 'I had amoxycillin for five days and now they've given me these stronger pills they say should shift the infection, but they don't seem to be doing anything. I'm not surprised – how are they supposed to diagnose you accurately over the phone? I'd hoped they'd help me at least a little, but ...'

'Put on your video so I can see you.'

I'm not ready for what I see when the grainy image depixelates. She looks exhausted. Her face is drawn and she has dark, puffy rings under her eyes.

'Can you take a look at my throat to see if it's inflamed?' she asks. Her thin voice crackles with each intake of breath. 'My eyesight isn't good enough and your dad's staying his distance just in case, even though we can't imagine how he wouldn't already have it if I do.'

She holds the phone to her face.

'Ma, that's your forehead, which looks fine, but you need to lower the phone so the camera points into your mouth. It's at the top.'

She finally shifts the camera to an angle that gives me a view of her tonsils.

I'm diagnosing my mother from 2,000 kilometres away over a video call.

'I don't see anything, Ma. It's a bit red, but that's all. I know you don't want to go near the hospital, but can't you just go into the surgery in Leven?'

'They're not seeing anyone. They're just redirecting people to the hospital. They have three phone numbers now: one for Covid, one for Covid-related problems – whatever those are – then 999. It took me two days to get through to my GP the first time I rang, and another two days the second time. They say I probably have some viral infection, but how are they to know? I thought it was Covid, then lung cancer, then—'

She's crying.

'I just can't stand the thought of leaving you and your sister and never seeing you again. You two are my world.'

'That's not gonna happen, Ma. You don't have any other symptoms besides the cough and sore throat. I'm sure if they suspected anything, they'd be doing more.'

'Oh, I'm not even angry with them. I know they've made a right mess of things and the Tories don't give a damn about us, but it's not that. I'm just upset that the whole thing's even happening. It beggars belief.'

With very few exceptions, no government is going to come out of this looking at all good. The news from Lombardy today is as damning as any of the British or US governments' missteps in the run-up to lockdown. A story in *La Repubblica* reported on a feature of the Lombardy region's containment strategy I'd somehow missed – the decision to place patients with coronavirus in care homes for the elderly, a policy that, in the last six weeks, has seen the death from the virus of a suspected 6,000 elderly residents. Attilio Fontana, the region's president, has attempted to shift blame onto the medical advisers and even the care homes themselves.

Lockdown Day 42

Italy will reopen in stages and by zone, according to the number of positive cases. We are in the dark about when 'Phase 2' will begin in Lombardy. The end date of quarantine stipulated in the latest decree is 3 May, but every political party, region and layer of government wants to do things their own way and is throwing in their two cents' worth, leaving us rich in opinions and speculation but poor in decisions.

It's all very Italian. In my days as a teacher, we'd have meetings to decide when we'd have our future meetings. To use the photocopier, we had to ask a receptionist to ask the janitor, who'd then come and do the photocopying for us. In my lessons with adult students, many a half-hour was lost to convoluted, circling discussions about where to have our Christmas or end-of-year pizza, or even our post-class *aperitivo*. B cannot be reached from A without first visiting every other letter in the alphabet.

The national mood is edgy. Anger's not far behind. As nations like Germany, Norway and even Spain begin making carefully detailed plans for lifting restrictions, we're mired in uncertainty. As far as I know, the restrictions here are the most extreme in the world, and yet the results have been less encouraging. This, too, is very Italian – the imposition of the most punitive controls in the expectation that a large percentage of the population will disobey. The rate of taxation here is among the highest in Europe, and yet the country remains chronically short of funds and tax evasion is more widespread than in any other nation in the European Union. While in the UK, Germany and even New York City restrictions allow people to go for a walk or exercise, here we have been stuck inside our homes for almost forty days without being allowed further than 200 metres from our front doors, and only if we happen to have young children or dogs.

Overnight, a giant hand-painted sign has appeared on one of the roads above town: 'CLOSE THE SUPERMARKETS, OPEN THE FORESTS.' I agree – surely there's less chance of contagion walking alone in a forest than standing in a queue fifty-people deep, even at a distance of two metres, outside (or inside) a supermarket. By the time I've hauled myself out of bed around noon, the sign's gone viral.

I meet Giuseppina soon after finishing the coffee I need to drink alone to prepare me for our coffee together.

'You look washed out again,' she tells me, peering over the balcony. 'Did you sleep?'

'Yes,' I say. 'I slept okay. I'm just recovering from all those days of work. I'll be okay soon.'

'If you need me, we can do the reverse of the walking-stick trick – instead of me battering on the floor with my stick, you can hit the ceiling with your broom or mop or whatever you have. Okay?'

'Thank you.'

'What did I tell you about thank-yous?'

She stands up from her chair and starts making her way down the stairs.

'I was meaning to ask you something,' she says. 'Over there, by the fence, there's a plant that should be coming into bloom soon. An azalea. It was Domenico's favourite. He saw it on the television, on a golf course somewhere in America. He never knew a thing about golf but he was besotted with these particular flowers, so he asked and asked until he found the name. Then he bought one and planted it there. It was the only time he ever showed any interest in plants. Come.'

I follow her along the top tier of the garden to a skeletal, budding bush. I had no idea it was an azalea.

'Now, these are beautiful things when they're in bloom, but there's something in them, some chemical or other. In the pollen, I think. You should ask your girl; the Turks feed their bees on it to make medicine and suchlike. Anyway, it gives me terrible allergies so I can't go anywhere near it. But it needs to be carefully looked after. If it gets too little water, it will shrivel up and die. If it gets too much water, the roots start to rot and the leaves all turn yellow and fall off. And on hot days it needs to be covered with a towel or a sheet for a few hours to make sure it doesn't get too much sun. Do you think you can help? With the gardener not coming and the girls busy most days, I'm afraid it will die. I know it's a hassle, but—'

'Of course I can.'

'*Grazie*, Kieran. I wouldn't bother you, but it was important to Domenico. And I'll pay you, of course, in bresaola.'

I'm back in bed by 3 p.m. and determined to stay there

until tomorrow. I send Aiyla a text telling her I'll call in the morning, pull down the shutters, and say goodbye to Lockdown Day 42.

Lockdown Day 43

Rain today. The sweetness crept in the window and filled my bedroom by the time I woke. Whoever said that people don't like change had never spent forty-three days in quarantine. I can't rouse myself to leave my bed, but knowing that when I finally do the view from my window will be different, however marginally, is more thrilling than even the arrival of spring; more thrilling even than the first snows of the year, signalling the beginning of the ice-climbing and ski-mountaineering season. I text Ma again before checking the news. She seems better, though she still has no clue if she has the virus.

People are starting to talk about reopening, about the end of quarantine. Different Italian regions want to stagger the loosening of restrictions, allowing the least affected to reopen on 4 May while the worst – Lombardy and Marche – will extend their lockdowns.

All this talk of reopening gets me thinking about the months ahead. From this angle, the future seems impossible. Maybe it's because the future that arrives will be entirely different to the one I imagined a few months ago, or perhaps this turn through the lower half of my condition's cycle is colouring my perspective, but I can't see the door. Does the fact of a door not leading to where you want amount to the door's absence? It feels like it. In the pre-coronavirus world,

I'd found a balance after decades of yo-yoing between the extremes of drab routine and shiftless itineracy. I'd seen scope for continuing a watered-down version of my nomadic existence, with Aiyla as the vital ingredient of stability and human connection my life had lacked. But now, it seems, there's no saying how long the curbs on going anywhere will remain in place. Months? Years? If so, bouncing back and forth between Sondrio, Fife, Istanbul and Brooklyn won't be an option.

It's 2 p.m. and I'm still in bed. I can hear Giuseppina upstairs, busying herself with cleaning. The rain's abated, but a thin drizzle gets thrown against my window every few minutes. With hindsight, I can now have little doubt that I was manic in the few weeks before this recent downturn – moderately so, but enough to make me worry about my own second wave. The depressive spells are usually shorter than the manic ones, meaning that if I don't level off in the coming days, sometime around the end of the week, I can probably expect the mania back with interest.

I'd hoped one of Holly's doctor friends might have been able to help, but I haven't heard back from her. All of them, I'd imagine, work in the public sector and can't just lay their hands on potent mood stabilisers without going through the proper channels.

Ma calls before I've managed to get out of bed. Her intuition needs few clues to detect the onset of an episode, so I think twice about answering, but know I'd suffer two minutes of hell until she replied to a text wondering if she's okay.

'I'm better,' she says when I answer. She sounds better, if only marginally. 'We thought we were short on a few things, so we used the ASDA website and got a delivery, and we've been upstairs washing it all for the past two hours. We ferried it all down to the kitchen then realised we don't know what half the frozen stuff is or how to cook it because there's no packaging left. Why aren't you speaking? Let me hear your voice.'

'I'm here, Ma. I'm just listening to you.'

'Are you managing to get enough to eat? I know Italy's a little behind the UK with home deliveries and technology and suchlike.'

'I'm fine. And we're not so far behind, Ma. We have online ordering and all that, they're just limiting it to people who need it most – you have to be over sixty-five to place an order and get delivery.'

'You sound tired. And you were stressed last week, I could see it. Are you sleeping okay?'

'Yep. I've just been working a lot.'

'Sure?'

'Sure.'

'Okay, well, I'll let you get back to it. And let me know if you need those pills – your dad seems hell-bent on getting out of here at every possible opportunity, so I may as well send him to the postal van.'

'I will.'

'You would tell us, wouldn't you, if there was something, you know ... not right?'

'Of course I would, Ma.'

'It's just that I know you try to protect us by keeping it to yourself, and it kills me to think you'd have to go through anything alone.'

Edinburgh, 1999

I trudged into the doctor's office in the Old Town an hour before my first lecture. I tried to avoid these places – the ones I couldn't easily excuse myself from if the need arose. It'd been happening more in the past few years: the need to escape; the itchy, jittery feeling that consumed me for weeks at a time and required a few hours of daily exercise to appease. Today, at least, it would be over in ten minutes, tops. I suffered from depression, had done since I was around fourteen, and was just meeting my doctor for a blether about how I'd been getting on with my medication.

The secretary led me into Dr Green's office and I sat opposite him while he thumbed through his notes. *Secretary*, I thought. *Secret*-ary. The keeper of secrets, derived from the Latin *secretus*, derived from—

'Kieran?'

Dr Green was leaning over his desk, his expression more serious than before I'd zoned out.

That was happening more those days, too – whenever I felt out of my comfort zone. Mental fugues: descents into the abstract world of words to avoid the undesirable reality of raw experience. There was something grounding in their logic, something comforting in their removal from the immediate.

Street sounds filtered in through the window: the heavy sigh of buses arriving and departing, people barking orders at the coffee kiosk outside the office entrance. That was another new thing – how sensitive I'd become to normally inoffensive noises in the space of just a few months.

'Kieran?' Dr Green repeated, his eyes fixed on mine with an unsettlingly earnest, tender gaze.

'Yeah, sorry.'

'Do you know what that means?'

I'd missed something, it seemed.

'What *what* means?'

'Bipolar.'

Bipolar. Bi. Polar. Two poles.

'Bipolar?'

'Yes,' he said, sliding a leaflet across the table. 'You might have heard "manic-depressive".'

Manic. Depressive.

The 'depressive' part was familiar, but the 'manic' bit sounded just a little too close to 'maniac' for comfort.

I left the leaflet on the table. As I stooped to read the cover, something clicked.

'Is that,' I said, 'what Howard Hughes had?'

Dr Green scrunched his nose.

'No, I don't think so. Bipolar is best understood as . . .'

He continued speaking, but I was lost in the leaflet. The rows of stolid bullet points glowered up at me with an unshakable stare. The picture of a friendly-looking doctor and a serenely grinning patient did little to warm the very clinical, cold matter-of-factness of the thing. It looked serious.

'Is it serious? I mean, is it . . . bad?' I asked, interrupting him. I'd been there more than ten minutes. I wanted to leave.

'It's like any illness. It has varying levels of severity. But the experiences you've described to me and your previous doctor – and your episode last month, of course – would suggest that we may have more success treating you for this rather than just depression.'

In 1999 there was no Wikipedia. Someone had tried to teach me about the internet in freshers' week but I'd lost interest quickly. We had books, after all. And leaflets . . .

I spent most of the following weeks in my dorm room, feeling as though I'd been possessed by some silent, invisible and unlocatable demon who'd gatecrashed my very existence.

Should I tell Ma? Pa? Cath? Nah, I thought, definitely not. They had enough going on. Besides, this wasn't the kind of news you ever wanted to give your family.

When I'd had my first depressive episodes, I'd needed Ma or Pa to be with me at all times. They'd follow me from room to room around the house, come with me on dinner-time walks in the woods behind town, ferry me everywhere by car to avoid leaving as little as a two-minute window in which the thoughts that lured me into the painful place within the painful place might reappear. I remember one morning, when I'd been this way for weeks, I woke early and the thoughts had woken with me. An infestation. The more you swat at them, the more you aggravate them and compel them to sting. I'd gone to Ma and Pa's room to wake them, but found them sound asleep, long after they'd normally have risen. Looking at them then, I realised for the first time the toll that my illness – that *I* – was taking on them. What was happening to me was, by proxy, also happening to them. I closed the door gently behind me and tiptoed downstairs.

Just like then, I decided that morning in Edinburgh, the only decent thing to do was to let them sleep.

The prospectus for the year ahead quickly edited itself into something altogether less appealing than I'd envisaged. There'd be fewer parties, probably. More doctor's visits. I guessed I'd have to forget about that girl I'd pulled a few times in the union, too. What if she saw it? And the lads ... Emotions and feelings and moods and all that just wasn't how we rolled. I'd also started writing for a magazine a few weeks previously. Should I stop that? Did crazy come across on the page, too?

Six months passed. The demon hadn't shown. I made friends. Lots of them. I liked them. They liked me. They didn't seem to think I was a maniac, nor did I feel I had any maniacal tendencies towards them, or anyone else for that matter. I'd been taking the meds the doctor had given me but felt like I was living in a world composed of glue. I couldn't go out any more, couldn't concentrate on papers, jogged like an octogenarian, spoke like Eeyore, climbed like a numpty any time I ventured up to Salisbury crags to play around in the old quarry.

I stopped taking the meds, and by late spring I'd stopped going to see the psychiatrist to whom I'd been referred by Dr Green. His office rang a few times and sent a few letters, but by then I'd convinced myself they'd been wrong. In a few weeks it would be summer. I'd be home, safe and happy for a month, and then on my way to America for an exchange year, thousands of miles away from anyone who knew my secret. Maybe there, I thought, it would just disappear.

It didn't just disappear.

The symptoms worsened. A series of colourful manic episodes landed me in hospital four times – once each in Arizona and California, two more back in the UK – and earned me a

$1,000 fine and night in jail for disorderly conduct in the town of Alamosa, Colorado. I moved to Portugal to teach and study for a PhD. There, my diagnosis was upgraded from Bipolar 2 to Bipolar 1, courtesy of my episodes' severity having officially crossed the threshold between hypomanic and fully-fledged manic somewhere between setting off on an early-hours jog along the beach and waking up in a Lisbon hospital two days later. Over the next few years, I overdosed on meds twice (accidentally – I was self-medicating and upping my dosage as circumstances and mood required until an overdose was inevitable) and ended up abandoning my PhD six months from completion, quitting my job and setting off on a year-long stint of aimless wandering and hitch-hiking around the US, where I sat out further hostilities in a commune in the mountains of New Mexico and in my tent in a lonely corner of Utah's Canyonlands National Park.

I'd hoped, I suppose, that a kind of exposure therapy would allow me, in time, to build up a form of resistance to whatever Bipolar might throw at me; that fine-tuning and doubling down on coping strategies would eventually yield results. But it didn't work out that way.

Still, I told no one barring my high-school girlfriend, who by then was living in Australia and who I'd made swear to secrecy. I had friends who had depression, so I could talk about that, but 'Bipolar' seemed too 'out there' for sharing. And as my awareness of the onset of episodes grew, I became increasingly expert at hiding my condition, reinforcing my suspicion that I'd never be 'found out' as long as I simply kept it to myself and never stuck around anywhere long enough for anyone to ask.

Fourteen years later, I'd lived in seven countries and five US states, and repeated the same process I'd gone through in Edinburgh nearly as many times, always convincing myself that a change of the outward would engender a change of the inward. Then an email arrived in my inbox while I was working on a tree farm in Scotland, having gone home to recover from a particularly crippling episode the previous year: *'Re: Teaching Position: Sondrio'*.

I knew I'd go before I'd even read through the details, but I also knew that this time I couldn't do it alone. This first extended stint at home since uni had taught me that: though I'd shielded my family from witnessing the worst of my condition's manifestations by staying away all those years, I'd also deprived myself of their support, which by then I'd learned was paramount to coping with those manifestations and all the associated day-to-day maintenance of life with Bipolar 1.

By then I'd also learned enough about the logistics of caring to understand that keeping it a secret wasn't doing them a favour, but perhaps the greatest harm any loved one can do to another. Caring, and all that it entails – worry, hurt, sleeplessness, anguish – is a right bestowed solely by someone's willingness to do it when fully apprised of the need. If someone's willing to do it for you, there's a moral imperative to let them.

The day before leaving for Sondrio, I was up in my childhood bedroom finishing off my packing. I could hear Ma and Pa downstairs, going about their business. Pa was fishing out old guidebooks for the Alps and tidying his climbing cupboard. Ma was singing a Barbra Streisand song while ironing my socks and boxers for the trip and squeezing things into my luggage that I'd already told her I didn't need – paracetamol, hand warmers, a microwavable egg poacher, around a kilo of shortbread biscuits – and wouldn't discover until unpacking two days later.

I knew then that their tomorrow could go one of two very different ways; that the words I'd been rehearsing in my head all morning would land at their door either a cause of all causes to rally round, or further evidence of life's inexorable unkindness. Either way, the fact that I would be the source of the inevitable hurt entailed in each eventuality made me nauseous.

Ma appeared in my room while I was thinking things through, semi-subconsciously dragging things out so there'd be no suitable moment to do the telling and I'd have to save it for the next visit, just as I'd already done a dozen times before.

'Mum,' I said, while she was folding my underwear into a neat bundle atop my bulging rucksack, 'I have something to tell you before I go.'

Her smile quickly capsized as she turned to face me.

'Is something wrong?'

'No,' I said. 'Well, yes, kinda, but—'

'I'll get your dad,' she said, somehow sensing the gravity of what was coming before I'd even offered an explanation.

We convened around the kitchen table, where nobody ever sat except for Christmas dinners or 'wee words'. It was the first time we'd sat there since I'd been busted skipping school at sixteen.

I skipped the pre-scripted spiel of preliminaries I'd been rehearsing in my room throughout the morning and blurted it out.

'I'm, eh, Bipolar,' I said.

Behind me, an imaginary jury gasped.

In front of me, Ma and Pa froze, Pa's teacup suspended mid-swig.

I had to look away from them to get the rest out, fixing my eyes on the carpet while reciting a stilted, automaton synopsis of everything I'd kept in their blind spot that last decade and a half: how long I'd had it, the original diagnosis, the hospitalisations, the love–hate relationship with meds, the shady justifications behind my reasons for keeping it secret so long.

Pa put his cup down on the table, then reached over and placed a hand on my shoulder. Ma swooped in for a hug. When I'd freed myself and finally looked up, both were smiling through their tears.

'There's no need to cry,' I said. 'It's not terminal or anything. It's just an illness—'

'That you've been living with all this time,' said Ma, clasping my hands, 'all on your own. We always knew there was something, well ... not quite right. We're not upset because of what it is, but because it's a *relief*.'

It sounded like she'd said 'a relief'.

'A ... *relief*?'

'Well, yes, a lot of things make sense now.'

Pa, whose eyes hadn't left me, nodded in agreement.

'We're proud of you, son,' he said.

Of all the sentiments I'd assumed the news might educe, pride was probably the last of them.

'You've lived a life most people dream of, and you've done it all with this ... horrible sickness.'

'Yes,' said Ma, squeezing my hand. 'And now that we know, we'll do whatever it takes to get you right and get the help you need. Things will get better now.'

I spent the rest of the day and the morning before my flight dodging hugs (Ma) and shoulder-rubs (Pa) as I finished the last of my packing. Emboldened by their response, I set aside a few hours to call my sister, Bob and my closest friends from uni, Adam and Cecilia, to tell them, too. Their reactions were nearly identical to Ma and Pa's: relief, understanding, pledges of support, and a confession that the confession was more of a corroboration of long-held suspicions. I shouldn't, with hindsight, have expected anything less. They were the ones who'd been there when my condition was nameless, so it stood to reason that their understanding would only amplify with an explanation.

Ma's prediction was right. Things did get better. Across the board. We'd always been close but, despite spending most of my time a few thousand kilometres away, in the years since that day we've only become even closer, as if, by telling them, I'd not been putting anything 'out there' so much as eliminating the only barrier that had ever stood between us. The next day, the hollow, sunken-tummy feeling that always appeared somewhere on the drive to the airport didn't come. Instead, when we said our farewells at the gate and I took my first steps into yet another unknown, I felt armoured, tooled up, underpinned by a pair of immovable ballasts that would steady and support every other step I took from then onwards. In the space of a few words, I'd gone from taking on life free-solo to taking it on with the protection of a fail-safe rope.

There's a knock at my door after Ma's call.

It's Giuseppina. She's wearing a mask.

'Excuse me for wearing this thing but I thought, with all the girls visiting me, I'd better keep it on in case I infect you with the virus. I don't have any of the symptoms, but they tell me you can have it without being sick. Fancy!'

I grab my own mask from the shelf by the door and put it on.

'Great!' she says. 'Now we can go to Banca Popolare with that scythe of yours and top up my pension and get the funds for your house in the mountains.'

'I'm in!'

'I was wondering if you might nip to the shop for me? The girls can't today and I've run out of flour. I should have asked them yesterday but it slipped my mind.'

I put on my shoes and head down Via Scarpatetti in my pyjamas and mask. There's a little square at the bottom of the street, surrounded on all sides by three-storey apartment buildings, some of them adorned with panels of faded frescoes and elaborate cornicing, and a shoebox of a grocery store. The store is run by Vittorio, who lives in the apartment above it with his wife and mother.

'*Ueilà!*' he says as I enter. 'I haven't seen you in ages.'

He's behind the glass cheese-and-meat counter, wearing his usual flour-stained blue apron and a huge, homemade mask that leaves only his smiling eyes and perfectly bald head visible.

I used to see him all the time when I worked at the language school. On nights when I finished early, I'd pass the shop on the way home and always find him at the service door, smoking and checking his phone. Each time, I'd join him for a smoke and we'd talk about Brexit, whisky or football, and he'd school me in the ways of the Mafia and the government's corruption, and remind me that southern Italians were a different species.

'Been busy,' I reply, not wishing to admit that I'd been shopping in the larger, cheaper supermarket on the edge of town.

'How are things up your way? Where your parents live?'

'Pretty much the same as here.'

'They locked up, too?'

'Yeah, but they're allowed out for exercise once a day, so it's not so bad.'

'I remember your mother. She was in here every day buying stuff for her cakes – those round things with the cream and jam inside. She brought some to me. Good, they were! She would continue speaking in English all the time even though I don't understand a word. She okay?'

'She's fine. Still making scones. She's a one-woman bakery.'

'Well, we all have to do something. I count my lucky stars that I'm a greengrocer – never thought I'd see that day. The restrictions here are too tough – everyone's gonna be in the *manicomio* [mental asylum] soon, never mind the hospital. How's their economy going to look then, eh? I'm praying they ease up after 4 May so we can at least leave the house for a walk, but who knows.'

'Yeah, I was trying to make sense of it from the papers this morning but they all say different things.'

'Don't read the papers! They're all full of shit. The trouble is those *giornalisti di merda* ... they have to fill their pages so they write whatever the hell they want. Journalists belong to the same class as politicians – corrupt, liars and unable to say a thing without an agenda.'

He hands me my bag of flour. I tell him to keep the change.

'Stop by when this is all over and we'll have a smoke together like the old days,' he says as I'm leaving.

'I don't smoke any more.'

'Ah, too bad,' he says, with no trace of sarcasm. 'Where have you been, anyway? Are you still at the school?'

'Nah. I quit a while back.'

'Ah, good. No more of those late finishes, eh? What are you doing now?'

'I'm a journalist.'

I do a quick traverse of the Scorpion Wall and check on the azalea before having dinner at 5 p.m., bringing it forward a few hours to see off another day. Before turning off my phone I call Aiyla and then check the news, hoping for better tidings, some sign that there won't be too many more days like this before we're done.

Lockdown Day 44

The heaviness has lifted. Only slightly, but instead of lying in bed until noon or later, I'm up at 8 a.m. and attempting to put in a few hours' work, even though my brain is dragging its heels.

During a break, I take out the yellow pocket diary I carry with me everywhere – number forty-five in a series I began keeping in my twenties, around the time of the earliest of the entries I read to Aiyla in week two of lockdown. Inside the back page of every volume I copy out an eight-point list of things to remember when it starts looking like the shit's headed in the direction of the fan:

1. Routine
2. Meditate
3. Exercise
4. Get out
5. Help others
6. Talk
7. Accept
8. They're feelings, not facts

Until I can get my hands on meds, these coping mechanisms are the only things standing between normal me and meltdown, so I'll have to use them fully.

Before I can figure out how the list might be customised to the rigours of lockdown, Enzo texts: *'I heard from my policeman friend. He says the police arrive only at 10 a.m. to stop people leaving town. If you want to go to the cheap supermarket, leave early and you'll be safe.'*

I'm out the door with a fistful of shopping bags in less than a minute. Yesterday, I checked my supplies and found that I'll be enjoying dinners of chickpeas and sweetcorn for the next week unless I manage to summon the courage for another supermarket visit. Also, shopping in the little supermarket in town is blowing my quarantine savings plan. All the work I've done this month has given me a little bit of financial leeway for the first time in my freelancing career, but I'll have a lot of hugs to give when this thing ends and the people who'll be receiving them all live on the far end of an expensive flight.

The roads and streets in town are busier than I'd expected and the car park at the supermarket already has a queue of five people, even though it won't open for ten minutes.

I get out of the car to stretch my legs and wander down to the edge of the car park, from where I can see the Sassella climbing crag, a 100-metre bluff of flaky, polished schist. Nicknamed *La Mediocre* by my climbing companions, the crag is avoided by most serious climbers in the valley because of its proximity to the road, poorer quality of rock and lack of more challenging climbs. At this moment, however, the glimmering schist is purest porn for my rock-starved eyes. *Just a ten-minute scramble*, I think . . . but a police car is parked at the entrance to the car park, one officer questioning a lady in a large camper van while another eyes me suspiciously, wondering why I've been standing there so long.

When a masked and rubber-gloved worker finally opens up the supermarket, I rush around and collect another two weeks' worth of food without incident. However, it seems Italians have finally started panic-buying. I'd hoped to buy some flour to make a batch of scones, but the shelf is barren. I ask one of the shop assistants if they have any in stock.

'Not a single bag,' she tells me. 'We sold out last week and don't expect to have any more until this is over.'

The items deemed essential purchases in times of crisis by the British and Italians respectively are very telling. In Britain, I'm told, the shelves stocking pasta, rice, toilet paper and tinned corned beef have been ransacked. People shopped as if they'd arrived in longboats. Here, every shopper is a connoisseur, in good times and bad. I see a woman lift and squeeze an aubergine to test for firmness. There is a queue of four at the fresh pasta counter. The tinned foods section remains fully stocked. The national prioritisation of quality over quantity remains. The market value of toilet paper is the same as ever. Most of those around me would rather starve than suffer a mediocre meal, reminding me of the Italian mountaineers of yore, who, in the lean years of the early twentieth century, had their porters schlep literal tons of cognac, champagne and fine claret up to lofty base camps in the Karakorum. Even the social media posts of home cooking and baking reveal a culinary schism between my two homelands, with Italian posters displaying elegant pasta dishes, daintily crafted desserts and pastries, and steaming piles of polenta, while my fellow Brits appear to be subsisting on banana bread and sourdoughs alone.

Driving home, I feel like I've pulled off a heist but decide to avoid shopping there in future. The sight of the crag, mediocre as it may be, was torturous, mostly due to knowing how much even a middling climbing session could help to stabilise my mood and see me safely through to the end of lockdown.

Aiyla calls while I'm showering my groceries.

She's dressed in an old hoodie, surgical mask and rubber dishwashing gloves. Her neighbourhood is full of stray cats and dogs, and over the past week she's been patrolling it with tins of food and water trays made from used ice-cream tubs, feeding whatever needs feeding. I love her.

'I'd love you more, though, if you didn't feel the need to wipe out my phone's storage space with a million photos of every moggie in Istanbul every day,' I say.

'Just trying to cheer you up a little bit, grumpy.'

'Yeah, I know.'

I tell her about my plan to double down on coping strategies.

'What's something you've always wanted to do that you can do at home?' she asks.

'I dunno ... Learn the piano, maybe? Or moonwalk? But I don't have a piano and—'

'You're the world's worst dancer.'

'Precisely.'

'Remember your Nietzsche – having a clear "why" helping you survive any "how", and all that.'

'It just feels like all my grand plans for the time in quarantine have kinda fallen by the wayside. I thought about resurrecting the book of poems I was working on last year but I'm pretty sure they're better off dead. The deckchair idea was great until I remembered I have no wood and zero carpentry skills. And I can't paint the house because I don't have any paint. I checked in the supermarket today in those centre aisles where they keep all the random stuff but their supply team are either Luddites who have no idea what's happening or just the most optimistic people on the planet – all they had were fishing rods and hiking clothes and barbecue stuff.'

'You're a climber. So ... climb.'

'This, coming from Miss You-Only-Ever-Think-About-Climbing-and-Not-About-Me?'

'Yes! Can't promise I'll make a habit of it, but for now you have my unconditional blessing.'

'I've been climbing. A lot. But the walls are kinda easy. They're great for a bit of exercise, and fuck knows how I would have managed without them, but there's no challenge, not really. I'm gonna be climbing like a newbie by the time this is over if I don't get any real practice in soon. I need to do more. You know, if I slept during the day and left here around midnight, I could get to the Masso di Arquino or Sassella and put in a few hours every night and nobody would ever know. And that way I could get in some real prep for the alpine climbing season and all the routes I'd planned on doing this summer, assuming we're open by then.'

She's looking at me the way mothers look at children with scraped knees or sub-par report cards, a look composed of two parts exasperation, one part pity.

'I get the feeling you're not gonna be my cheerleader on this one,' I say.

'Not exactly.' She shakes her head. 'I don't get it. Why this? Why now? You've been doing fine.'

'I *was* doing fine, yeah. But you were right last week. I feel something happening. I think I'm, eh ... "cycling".'

'I know.'

'You know?'

'Of course I know. I'm a psychologist, dipshit.'

'Ah, true.'

'Look, I know you need to do exercise to flush out your headshit, and it's good that you're trying to give yourself something to build towards, but that wasn't what I had in mind. I also think it might be helpful to try a little change of perspective, too.'

'Go on.'

'You have to remember why you're a climber.'

'The genetic, Pa-gave-me-this-and-my-big-nose origin theory or the because-it's-better-than-sex-and-cannoli origin theory?'

'None of the above ...'

'Then what?'

'Because it keeps you sane.'

'That's a good answer too,' I say, slightly scorned, 'but I don't see how it rules out night-time sessions in Arquino or Sassella.'

'Have you heard of Maslow's Hierarchy of Needs?'

'Heard about it, yeah. Have a clue what it's about? No.'

'It's a motivational theory of need fulfilment. He sees our needs as a pyramid. At the bottom, there are more basic, phys-iological needs – food, water, warmth, rest, safety – and higher up more advanced needs like relationships and accomplishment and creativity and self-actualisation. In the hierarchy, you have to satisfy the lower levels before you can go up. This crisis has landed us all back at rock bottom, so we should all just be focusing on our most basic needs – it's unrealistic to expect to do more. You just have to keep yourself safe and sane, and ride it out before you can start thinking about doing anything else.'

'Where does your cat salvation programme fall into this? And Nietzsche? And my need for a project to work on?'

'With the cats, I'm taking care of the basic physiological needs of others while squeezing in a bit of socialising – kinda – and getting a glimpse of achievement for myself.'

'And Nietzsche?'

'It's like you've always said – helping others is the best way to help yourself. You're doing that just by staying home – for you, your family, for Giuseppina and her family, for me and for the community as a whole. *We're your why.* That's how this works. *Surviving for us* is your lockdown project, and you're succeeding. Italy has had the longest and strictest lockdown outside of China, for fuck's sake, and you've been doing well. Acknowledge that. And don't fold now – the end is so near.'

'What about climbing?'

'Well, it's just like Giuseppina told you when she was talk-ing about how things were when she was young. You have to do everything you can with the resources at *your* disposal to keep yourself psychologically fit enough to do the first part. It's not in any of the professional literature, sure, but for you that means using the tools and strategies that you've developed over the years that you know work, i.e. climbing. Now's not the time to be branching out and broadening your horizons. It's time to be doing watered-down versions of the things that make life tolerable the rest of the time, doing whatever works. The reason you're getting so frustrated is because you're trying to do Maslow's stage three, when one and two aren't covered.'

'Okay, so, just so we're clear: you're not only giving me your blessing to climb as much as I want but actively prescribing it as a member of the psychological community who has finally come to see the light?'

'Something like that . . .'

Lockdown Day 45

I wake at 4 a.m. Before I've even opened my eyes, I know the depressive spell has gone and I've looped straight back into mania. It's a lighter shade of manic, a cherry-blossom pink vignetted by a flamingo-coloured border that may or may not dim into darker hues in the days ahead.

The next two hours do nothing to disprove the suspicion. In that time I finish my penultimate assignment for the month, do 200 push-ups, 200 sit-ups, bake a batch of scones and spend €300 on Amazon on stuff I'm not sure I really need: 50 surgical masks each for my sister and parents, a digital thermometer, a Turkish grammar book, new climbing shoes and two packs of climbing holds for Pa. I go outside for the first time in days without feeling the daylight and birdsong and the sound of my neighbours working in their gardens as an affront. If there was someone to dance with, I'd be dancing.

This is new territory for me – cycling so quickly. But the fact that I'm aware that I'm cycling quickly is probably the best indication that things aren't approaching critical just yet.

With most things in life, there is a kind of exposure therapy: the more you walk the terrain, the more you get to know it and the easier it becomes the next time around. While this is true of Bipolar to a certain extent, episodes are always new terrain. There are qualitative similarities and recurring features, but each one is a law unto itself as regards duration and intensity, and governed by a kind of integrated amnesia that obliterates the memory of those past, making self-awareness virtually impossible once they're fully underway.

Giuseppina's shutters rattle open behind me while I'm standing on the lawn drinking in the remnant musk of last night's rains and inspecting the flowers. She waves from the window and signals for me to wait.

While I'm waiting I take off my slippers and let the dewy grass tickle my feet. Giuseppina reappears a few minutes later with two espresso cups.

'*Buongiorno,*' she says, plodding down the stairs in her slippers and dressing gown, and leaving one of the cups on the landing by the front gate.

'*Buongiorno*, Giuseppina!' I call back, more emphatically than I'd intended. I add 'shouting' to 'shopping', 'racing thoughts' and 'excess energy' on the mental list of red flags I've sighted thus far.

'You look well today,' she says, edging herself into her chair with the aid of the banister, 'but you should put a shirt on. People will begin to say I have a toy boy if they see us out here every day with you dressed like that. Don't think those town gossips will be distracted by a little pandemic. Besides, you'll catch the *aria*.' Despite their seemingly innate hardiness, the Valtellinese are as fearful as other Italians of the evil doings of air, holding it accountable for not only chills and colds but also stiff necks, headaches, stomach aches, back pain and a litany of other ailments. My watch tells me it's 22 degrees outside and the draught is at least 20 miles per hour short of what would qualify as a 'wee breeze' in the Kingdom of Fife.

'I feel a bit better. Are you okay?'

She shrugs.

'Okay isn't the same as what it was, but I suppose the new version will have to do for now.'

I wander around to the front of the house after our coffee and do a few barefoot traverses of the Scorpion Wall. Before the depressive spell set in and robbed me of my strength, I was racking up around 750 metres of climbing per day. If what I think might be coming is actually coming, getting back up to that figure quickly is going to be key to getting through it unscathed.

In the afternoon, a text from one of my climbing friends arrives while I'm working. He and a few other regulars in our climbing circle have decided to petition the local government to ease restrictions on movement outside the town:

PETITION TO OPEN THE FORESTS

This petition to the Prefect of the Territorial Office of the Province of Sondrio requests a relaxation of restrictive measures related to outdoor activities.

In Valtellina we are a mountain people. We are used to fatigue and restrictions, manual labour, cold and loneliness, but not to live far from our woods, pastures and streams. A mountaineer locked in the house becomes ill in body and spirit.

We are fully aware of the seriousness of the ongoing epidemic. However, we believe that the measures to contain it should be appropriate to the territory and the population, and it does not make sense to take the rules enforced in high-density cities and simply apply them to the mountains.

Those who go to walk in the woods alone or with their family, who go to chop wood, to cultivate their vegetable garden or who bring their child to a meadow, cannot infect or be infected by anyone. These activities are the foundations of our daily life, and a forest is a much safer place from the virus than the supermarkets or offices where we are still allowed to go.

Please give us back our woods, our mountains, our land.

I've met very few Valtellinese who are not mountain-goers in some form. The mountains are to them – even to those who claim to have no appreciation for mountaineering or even hiking – what the sea is to the people in the villages dotted along the coast where I grew up in the East Neuk of Fife, what the Santa Ana winds are to the Californians, what the desert is to the Bedouins in the Levant and North Africa – not only a part of the landscape they occupy, but an indelible presence in the mental landscape. A Valtellinese friend who'd gone to work in London for a few years once told me that, while there, she could feel the mountains' absence all around her, even when she was indoors. It was the first thing she noticed when she woke up in the morning and would keep her awake at nights – the emptiness where the mountains should be. When she returned to the valley, it was as though they'd been waiting for her, she said, and she felt a strong sense of having betrayed something fundamental to her nature by staying away so long. I've felt this too. Anywhere else, there's a ghostly absence, an emptiness to any skyline not abbreviated by mountains. The lack of the protection they give from the rest of the world leaves a feeling of exposure, a longing for their womb-like embrace.

When I'm in bed, I remember the azalea. I put on my slippers and head outside to douse the base of the plant with a litre or two of water from the can I now keep on my terrace. When I return to my room, the notification light is flashing on my phone. It's a message from Pa.

'Your ma and me are missing you, lad. Just wanted to make sure you know that. You take care.'

He's still online.

'Miss you too, Dad,' I write.

'Aye, I suppose we'll get through all this, one way or another.'

'Couldn't sleep. Been watching a series about snow leopards. On episode four already. Ma went up to bed at about seven so been spared Coronation Street and usual baking guff. Think we might need to add Mongolia to my bucket list. Easier done than Denali at my age anyway.'

'Seven? Is she okay?'

'Aye. Just tired. Wearing herself out with her worrying as usual. Nowt to worry about. You doing okay?'

'Yep. Just waiting for this to be over. Reading guidebooks in quarantine = bad idea. Last time I salivated so much over a picture it was of a Spice Girl, circa 1993.'

'We'll have plenty of climbing to make up for when this is over, that's for sure.'

'Piz Badile in autumn, ATS permitting?'

'ATS?'

'All This Shite.'

'Aye.'

Lockdown Day 46

When I hear my phone ringing with her video call in the morning, I don't suspect anything. I've been up for hours and have lost track of time, putting in twenty-minute sprees of work between push-ups, pull-ups on the doorframe and moonwalk attempts across the kitchen floor. I glance at the clock and see it's 6 a.m., 5 a.m. UK time. When the image on the screen clears, I understand immediately. She's on the sofa in the living room in her dressing gown. Her eyes are bleary and cheeks a fiery scarlet. She's wiping tears from them while trying to speak, but each attempt produces only a mewl from her contorted mouth followed by a shrill wheezing sound.

'Ma? Ma, what's going on?'

Before she's even spoken, tears are streaming down my face. I know. I don't know how I know, but I know.

'I have it,' she says. 'The virus.'

My guts feel as though they'll drop through the floor. I stare at the screen, looking for the clue that will tell me it's a joke.

Nothing. Just my mother, sobbing and whimpering with

stuttered breaths in the living room of our family home, over 1,000 miles away.

My mother has Covid-19.

'Ma, no,' I whimper, my voice suddenly that of a child.

'Now, don't you get upset,' she says, palming tears from her cheeks. Her voice is croaky and thin. Every time she breathes in, her stuttering breath is punctuated by a squeal, like a rickety door blowing in the wind. 'I was up through the night and took my temperature. It was nearly 39. I've been having bother breathing, too, so I phoned the hospital and they're going to take me in today. When it was just the cough and the aches, we thought it might be something else, but the triage nurse I spoke to said . . .'

She tries to smile, but her breath catches in her throat, crackling like spitting embers. Her hair's grown long in the last month and parts of her fringe are stuck to her forehead. A few beads of sweat dot her upper lip.

My insides feel itchy. I'm rocking in my chair, trying to put out the fire in my skin.

'Don't you worry, darling,' she says. 'Nothing's going to happen to me. They'll take me in and sort me at the hospital, then I'll be back. And you'll be back soon, too, then we'll get along to St Andrews for coffee and finish the Fife Coastal Path like we said, eh?'

'Yep.'

'I need you to stay strong for Mum, okay? Don't get upset.'

I'm speaking to my mother on a 2x5-inch screen. She's 1,327 miles away. She's infected with a virus that's killed nearly a quarter of a million people.

It can't be real. It can't be real. It can't be real.

The arm of my chair breaks off in my hand. I let it drop to the floor, unable to look away from the screen. Ma's eyes loll drunkenly in her head, unable to focus. When she was speaking, there was the comfort of her voice, the semblance of normality. When she stops there's only the silence, punctuated by the wheezing every time she breathes in.

'Ma, where's Dad?' I ask, more to keep her speaking than anything else.

'He took the dog out,' she whispers, lifting her head towards the phone. 'They're on the beach.'

Ma's got coronavirus; Pa's on the beach with the dog.

'What the fuck is he doing on the beach?'

'No, don't be angry with him. He's been a gem. I sent him away. I was trying to call the hospital and then your aunty Brenda phoned. He was getting flustered so I told him the dog could do with a walk. He was—'

A gravelly cough cuts her off.

I let out a sob before I can smother it.

She sits forward in the chair and looks into the camera. 'Oh, I wish I could give you a cuddle.'

'You too, Ma.'

'Now, I should try the hospital again to see what they've arranged.'

'Use the house phone and leave our call open.'

She lifts the house phone from the table beside the chair and dials the hospital number. After a dozen rings, I hear a man's voice.

I can't believe how much the world has changed in the past ten minutes. When the phone rang, I'd been annoyed by the disruption so soon into my day. Now this.

After taking her details, the man asks Ma why she's calling.

'I've had this awful cough for weeks and then just last night my temperature went up and I started having difficulty breathing. I felt—'

Her voice breaks off. I hear her sobbing.

'I'm sorry,' she continues. 'I'm just worried and my children live so far away. My son's in Italy and my daughter's in New York. I couldn't bear not seeing them again.'

She coughs again. Her shoulders heave, shaking tears onto the collar of her dressing gown.

Two minutes later, she thanks the man for his help and ends the call.

'They're going to ring me back,' she says. 'He was just directing the calls. They're very busy, he says.'

'How are you feeling now?'

'I'm just so hot. My ears feel like they're on fire.'

'You have to keep your temperature down. Have you got a cold compress?'

'Yes, I had one this morning. I'll get it.'

I hear her feet scuffle on the living room carpet, then on the tiles on the kitchen floor, followed by the running of a tap.

'I did this a lot with you and your sister when you were wee,' she says when she returns to the living room. 'I haven't done it in years.'

She tilts her head back against the headrest, laying the wet tea towel across her brow.

'Now,' she says, letting her arms hang limp, one in her lap, the other over the side of the chair, 'there we go.'

A few minutes pass. I start taking screenshots. I don't know why. Desperation, probably. A way of grabbing onto her in the only way I can. There are thirty-second intervals when she seems to have fallen asleep but each one is interrupted by a bout of coughing that jolts her forward in the chair.

I hear the sound of cars passing at five-minute intervals outside her window; the wood pigeon in the neighbour's fir tree. Through the gap in the blinds I see our neighbour walking past with his dog.

'Do you think I should phone your sister?' Ma says after fifteen minutes. 'She'll be sleeping. She has a conference today, with Wall Street people, but I just want to see her.'

I dread the idea of spending the next few minutes out of contact but know my sister would never forgive me if I didn't let Ma call.

'Call her,' I say. 'And call me right back when you're done.'

I go to the drawer in the bathroom for my meds. Inside I find an empty prescription package and the ten packs of Lemsip that Ma had sent me after she'd failed to find it in any of Sondrio's pharmacies on her last visit.

I have no meds.

I stagger into the garden. My legs feel like they're about to give way. I steady myself against the wall, then lower myself to the ground, lie on the turf and begin sobbing. My body is juddering and spasming uncontrollably. The sound of my own whimpering is somehow distant, as if emanating from the depths of a cave, and not mine.

I must have been lying there for almost half an hour before I pick up my phone from the grass and call Aiyla.

When she answers, I try to speak but can't.

'Kieran? Kieran, baby, what's happening?'

'Mum,' I say. The rest of it won't come.

'Your mum? What happened? Take a deep breath.'

I take a deep breath.

'She has it,' I say. 'The virus.'

'Oh, fuck. How do you know it's the virus? I thought she was getting better.'

'She has the fever now. And difficulty breathing. It seems—' The words are stolen from my mouth before I can speak them.

'Just take a few deep breaths for me, okay?'

I close my eyes and focus, but my body is vibrating and each sob is like a punch, stealing away my breath before it's passed my throat.

'I should be there with her,' I finally manage to say.

'Your dad's there with her. He'll take care of her.'

'He's not. He's on the beach with the bloody dog. I could fucking kill him.'

'Don't say that. He—'

'Why not? She hasn't left the house in six weeks. If she has the virus it's because he brought it home.'

'Look, I'm sure he's been safe. There are tons of ways she could have got it. Listen to me. You've been manic recently. I know this is horrible, especially in these circumstances, but do you think you might be panicking more because of the way you've been feeling these past few days?'

'It's my mother, Aiyla. She has Covid, a virus that's killing tens of thousands of people every week.'

'And which hundreds of thousands are surviving every week, even when infected. You have to remember that, too.'

'I have to go,' I say, realising we've been on the phone for too long. 'I'll call later.'

I try calling Ma but her phone's engaged. Still on to Cath, probably. I go to my seat on the terrace and collapse into it, burying my head in my hands.

I cannot lose my mother.

I.

Cannot.

Lose.

My.

Mother.

I hear the jangling of the goats' bells in my neighbour's garden. A gaggle of birds is gibbering in the branches of the magnolia. The growl of my neighbour on the other side of the house starting up his mower sounds like a swarm of helicopters.

A mosquito lands on my knee. I watch dumbly as it tilts its head closer to the fabric of my pyjama trousers, bites me and flies off.

I get up from the chair and wander down to the grass at the front of the house. I try Ma's number again but she's still busy.

I walk back around to my front door. I am sobbing again. My breathing's shallow and jerky, my body simultaneously wired and overcome with a subaqueous sluggishness. When I reach the bottom of the steps on my terrace, I hear a voice on the street. A lady appears, speaking to someone on her phone as she passes the gate. She glances inside and stops when she sees me.

'*Signor*, are you okay?' she asks. She's wearing a hairnet and mask. I don't recognise her.

She says something into the phone then puts it away in her pocket.

'*Signor?*'

CLIMBING THE WALLS

She grabs one of the rungs of the gate with a rubber-gloved hand and leans in closer.

'My mother has the virus,' I say. My voice is guttural, unrecognisable, somehow guilty.

'*Santa Maria,*' she says. 'Is she inside, your mother?'

'No.'

'In the hospital?'

'No. She's in Scotland.'

'*Dio santo,*' she says, her eyes widening, then waves a hand towards the gate. 'Come here.'

I climb the five steps to the landing in front of the gate and slump against the wall beneath Giuseppina's bathroom window.

I look up at the woman. The skin on her forehead is wrinkled like a withered apple. Her eyes are a vibrant green. She lifts a hand to shield them from the sunlight and uses the other to tuck a curl of hair that has escaped her hairnet behind her ear.

There is static in my head. My t-shirt is soaked with tears and is clinging to my chest. I zone out for a moment and when I look back at the woman I realise she's been speaking.

'I'm sorry,' I say, 'I didn't understand.'

'Do you speak Italian?'

'Yes.'

'Your mother – is she with someone?'

'Yes. My father.'

'That's good. And you – do you have someone here with you?'

'No,' I say, 'I'm alone.'

'*O, Signore.* Do you have friends?'

'Yes. And my landlady. She lives upstairs.'

'Good,' she says, nodding her head. 'You mustn't be alone. Call her. Or one of your friends. Anyone. If you want, you can open the gate and I'll come inside.'

Something in her words dumbfounds me. I hear them, but they are just sound, devoid of meaning.

My phone rings. I scramble to my feet. It's Ma.

'Thank you,' I say to the lady. 'You've been very kind.'

'Sto preghando per voi' (I'm praying for you all), she says, and continues up the street.

I take the phone inside.

'Hi darling,' Ma says when I answer. 'Your dad's home. We're just deciding if I should go to the hospital. I'm stable enough now, I think, but if it gets any worse then I might have no choice. Do you want to speak to your dad?'

'No,' I say. 'Stay on the phone.'

I want to look at her. Why haven't I ever taken the time to sit and look and marvel at the woman who is my mother?

'I had a good day yesterday, and the day before,' she says, as a fresh tear spills over her puffy cheeks. 'I just don't understand why it's got worse overnight.'

The house phone rings again. It's her sister, my aunt Brenda. She passes her mobile to Pa.

'Try not to worry, son,' he says. 'If she has it, then she's had it for a long time and she's fought it off this far. That says a lot.'

I can't speak to him. I know my anger's irrational and misplaced, but he's the only target for it without a direct line to Westminster.

'You're obviously upset. Do you have anything you can take to help you? Medication, I mean?'

'I'll be fine, Dad. But I need you to take care of her. I fucking hate that I can't be there and I need you to be me until she gets better, okay?'

'Of course, son,' he says. 'I'm doing all I can.'

We sit in silence. I hear Ma explaining to my aunt what the hospital have told her. A fly buzzes around my kitchen. Through my window I hear someone hammering in the streets below and the screams of a child. The world hasn't stopped.

Ma returns a few minutes later, wiping her face.

'Now, just you go and do your normal things, darling. We'll wait and see what the hospital says and keep you updated. I'm very tired so I'm going back to bed to rest.'

'Okay, Ma.'

'I love you,' she says, touching her fingers against her flaking lips then pressing them to the screen.

'I love you too, Mum.'

I go outside and lie on the grass, hoping to see Giuseppina, but she doesn't come. After ten minutes, I go back inside, put on my trainers and a pair of shorts, and start running.

I sprint up the hill and take a left, running at full tilt first down the top of Via Scarpatetti and the staircase leading into a cobbled square on the edge of the *cittavecchia*, then over the bridge across the Mallero River and on to the back streets, avoiding the town centre. I glance at my phone to check for incoming calls or messages every thirty seconds as I continue down an empty residential street lined with apartment blocks. On the other side of the park, a potholed road leads along the front of a dozen or so large villas to the foot of the Sassella and Inferno vineyards, which occupy most of the hillside between the valley floor and the village of Triangia, some 500 metres above. I turn left at the end of the road onto the rough, cobbled *mulattiera* (mule path) that leads to the Santuario della Madonna della Sassella, the chapel where Domenico and Giuseppina got married, which stands on an isolated bluff looking down the valley in both directions, directly above the town bypass.

I stumble on a turn in the path, dropping the phone and scuffing my knee along the gritty surface. I check the phone's okay and continue. By now I've been running for around thirty minutes. My body is pulsing, but even charging at full speed is not enough to get out of me the seething anguish that's inside. I clench my fists and begin thumping my hands against my hips and stomach, as if the pain could be beaten out of me.

I call Ma as soon as I'm home. Pa answers.

'The hospital called,' he says. 'They offered to send an ambulance, but she wants to stay home. She's scared she won't be able to speak to you and your sister if she goes in. We spoke to her GP, too – Dr Thompson. She says all the symptoms suggest she probably has it, but she can't do the test unless we drive into the hospital in bloody Dunfermline. Anyway, she says that being able to speak on the phone is a good sign – most of the ones getting taken into the Covid ward can barely talk. I think staying home's the best thing to do. The NHS wasn't prepared for this and the hospitals are overrun. They're admitting thousands of new patients every day. Over a thousand people died yesterday, for Christ's sake. It's like Italy at the peak, back in late March, only Boris and Co. had plenty of forewarning and still just sat twiddling their thumbs.'

'Can I speak to her?'

'We should let her rest. Just go and keep yourself busy as best you can. I'll let you know if there's any change.'

'How can you be so calm?'

'Getting myself panicked is not going to help anyone, is it? Besides ...'

He cuts himself off.

'What?'

'Well, I didn't want to say it. I know this is hard for you, being so far away and with all those people dying over there, but I'm worried you're getting yourself too worked up when there might be nothing to worry about.'

I try to count to ten. When I get to three, I say:

'Dad ...'

'Look, I'm not criticising. I'm just saying that it seems like you're panicking and, well, there's a chance that you might be ... overreacting.'

One, two ...

'You mean like the last time I was overreacting?'

This isn't the first time I've faced the threat of losing one of my parents.

It was the end of my first year in Sondrio. Pa had come over for a summer climbing holiday and after a week of doing routes in Val di Mello and Valmalenco we'd decided to take on Piz Palü and Piz Bernina before he headed home.

We caught the last cable car up to the Diavolezza hut and bivouacked on the moraine at the foot of the Pers Glacier, at just under 3,000 metres. We were on our way by two the next morning, crossing the glacier south-eastwards before looping up through a steep, cascading maze of crevasses and seracs towards the first of the three peaks of Piz Palü.

We'd planned on doing the full traverse of all three

peaks, spending the night in the Marco e Rosa mountain hut, and then taking on Piz Bernina by the Italian route the next morning.

Well into his sixties, Pa had been able to keep up with me even when I was at my fittest and doing big mountains every weekend, but on visits home over the past few summers I'd noticed him slowing down. That morning, however, he was labouring more than usual. The snow had refrozen nicely overnight, so the snow bridges over the crevasses were solid and the going far easier than I'd expected, but Pa was pausing every few hundred yards to catch his breath and the rope between us coming taut every twenty or thirty steps while we were moving, forcing me to stop.

'I'm coming, I'm coming!' he'd shout. 'Old age doesn't come by itself, you know!'

We'd planned on reaching the hut by early afternoon, but by lunchtime we'd only just left the last of the three peaks. We still had the descent down to the saddle above the Fortezza Ridge and the long traverse below the Bellavista peaks and Piz Argient. The terrain there was notoriously riddled with deep crevasses covered by snow bridges, all of which the afternoon sun would be weakening with every minute that passed.

Just below the saddle, the rope went tight again.

'I think I'll need to take a breather,' Pa called after me.

We'd taken a breather no more than twenty minutes ago. I was worried about the weakening of the snow bridges in the midday heat and wanted to push on, but when I turned around Pa was already sitting in the snow, hunched over and gasping for breath.

I coiled in the rope as I walked back towards him.

He'd unzipped his jacket and taken his gloves off by the time I reached him and was rubbing the left side of his face.

'You okay, *Faither*?'

'Aye, grand,' he said, but his face had a pained expression and his whole body seemed to have stiffened. He was slumped awkwardly against the slope, not in a way that looked the least bit restful.

Just then he let out a groan and grabbed his side.

'What the fuck was that?' I said.

Another minute passed before he spoke. He was panting and had clenched his hand over his chest.

'Just indigestion, I think . . .' he said.

'You haven't eaten a thing all—'

He let out another groan.

'Alright, I'm phoning the helicopter.'

His eyes widened.

'Don't you dare! The same bloody thing happened on Monte Rosa in '92 and Mont Blanc a few years later. There's nothing to worry about – it's just the altitude.'

'We're only at 3,600 metres.'

'I'm not acclimatised. I've been stuck at sea level for the past five years!'

He convinced me not to make the call and just to let him rest up.

Another two hours passed. Then, without saying anything, he got to his feet.

'If you don't mind, we'll just head back down now.'

It was 2 a.m. by the time we got back to the car, 4 a.m. by the time we reached Sondrio.

As we parked up outside the apartment, Pa said, 'Please, don't ever tell your mother this happened.'

At 6 a.m. a noise in the kitchen woke me. I got up and found Pa in the living room packing his rucksack.

'Ready to go?' he said.

'Eh? Where?'

'I fancied this one,' he said, spreading out a map on my coffee table.

He pointed out a peak on the map – Pizzo Tresero, a 3,650-metre affair in the Ortles-Cevedale Group that I'd never done before but imagined would be no cakewalk.

'Dad, d'you think—'

'Please . . .' he said.

We set off twenty minutes later and ended up doing both Tresero and the taller, neighbouring Punta di San Matteo. We didn't talk about what had happened on Piz Palü – not that day on Pizzo Tresero or in the months before I returned home for Christmas. As far as I knew, there was no recurrence.

During the Christmas break we waited for a window of decent weather to do our last hill of the year. We chose Beinn a' Ghlò, an easy trio of tops just north of Pitlochry. It had been one of my first Munros when I was a kid and seemed ideal, given the worries I'd been harbouring about Pa's health.

'Dad,' I said on the drive up, 'I've been feeling a wee bit, eh, "up" these last few days, so I'm gonna jog up to the first top to get it out of my system, okay? Then I'll come back and join you and we can do the other two together.'

'Fine by me.'

We arrived at the trailhead at around 6 a.m. I left him at

the car park and hurried up to the first top, turning every so often to look for the glow of his headlamp on the snow in the darkness below.

It was almost light by the time I reached the first summit. The sky to the east was aglow, the rising sun a bloodshot eye searing beneath a low bank of cloud above Ben Vuirich and the rounded tops near Glenshee. To the north, the southern bulwark of the Cairngorms looked like the threshold of another world. To the south-west, I saw no sign of Pa.

I pulled on a jacket and took pictures of the sunrise before heading back down. The wind had kicked up suddenly just before I'd reached the summit and was now blowing me sideways with every step.

I expected to find Pa not far below the top. I'd spent at least fifteen minutes on the summit taking pictures and changing clothes, and my tracks in the snow would have saved him the trouble of breaking trail. But when I reached the edge of the small plateau around a third of the way down, he was nowhere to be seen. I continued downward and found him just below the halfway point.

'You okay?' I asked.

'Aye, just trying to get my breathing going,' he said without stopping. 'I've been getting slack these past few months and my lungs are wondering what's going on. You go on ahead; don't let my dithering ruin your day. You'll freeze your knackers off going at my pace, anyway.'

'Okay,' I said, eying him in search of any of the signs I'd seen on Piz Palü. 'But I'll loop back again soon.'

I jogged back up to the summit but this time turned back down immediately.

I found Pa not too much further on from where I'd left him and this time stayed with him until we reached the top, following behind as he plodded haltingly through the knee-deep snow. Just as we came to the stone shelter next to the summit, I heard a muffled groan through the wind.

'Dad, what's going on?' I said, grabbing him by the arm.

He didn't reply. He was rubbing his left shoulder and staring wide-eyed at the ground.

'Do you think we should go down?'

He didn't look up, but kept his eyes fixed on some point in the snow past my hip, his face frozen in a canted grimace.

'Aye, I think we'd maybe better.'

We stumbled a few hundred metres down the hill, retracing our steps. Seeing that Pa was limping and struggling to keep his balance, I grabbed him and threw his arm over my shoulders.

I'd expected him to resist, but he didn't say anything.

Below the plateau he came to a stop, shook himself free of my arm, and dropped to the snow.

I panicked, first dumping all of my rucksack's contents on the snow to find my phone and map, then sprinting up to a small hillock to scan the lower part of the hill for anyone who could help.

No one.

I ran back down to Pa, who hadn't moved.

'This time I'm phoning the helicopter,' I said.

'No!' he cried, panting. 'Don't be daft. Nobody gets a bloody helicopter off Beinn a' bloody Ghlò. We're ten minutes from the car.'

I looked down the hillside and located the forest where we'd parked the car. It couldn't have been much more than a mile, but even at our previous rate of progress I knew it would take at least an hour.

I phoned the chopper.

'Call them back and tell them I'm fine, for Christ's sake,' Pa said as soon as I'd hung up. Until then he'd been slurring his words, but now he seemed to be focusing all of his energies on getting his point across.

His chest heaved with a few deep breaths before he came out with it.

'You need to settle down,' he said. 'You're overreacting. You said yourself you were a wee bit up, didn't you?'

'Dad . . .'

'I'm just saying, you might not be seeing this clearly – it's happened before, mind?'

'What the fuck, Dad? I haven't been properly manic in months. And you're lying halfway up a hill in the snow having, what . . . a heart attack?'

We waited. I took off my jacket and wrapped it around Pa's shoulders then lay behind him to create a windbreak. We'd stopped on one of the most exposed patches of the hillside and the wind was throwing a steady shower of spindrift across the slope. I doubted a chopper would be able to land.

We waited.

After half an hour I called 999 again. The operator took our coordinates a second time, then told me to leave my phone on and wait for Mountain Rescue to call back.

Fifteen minutes later, the call hadn't come.

Every so often Pa would wince and clasp his chest. Between times, he lay still, his left shoulder arched awkwardly and face drooping on one side.

'I'm gonna run and get help,' I said, and set off before Pa could stop me.

Before I'd made it a hundred steps down the hill, I saw the helicopter on the horizon. I lurched back up again and reached Pa just as the winchman was descending.

'What an embarrassment,' Pa said, then closed his eyes as the winchman landed beside us and strapped him into the stretcher.

A minute later I was alone on the hillside.

When I found Pa's room at the hospital in Dundee, he was propped up on his bed and broke into a big, lopsided grin.

'A minor stroke, we think,' the nurse said, 'but we're waiting for the scan results to determine exactly what happened. The next few hours are critical, but there's no need to worry. He's in good hands.'

Pa reached over the bars on the bed and tugged my hand.

'Told you you were overreacting,' he said.

I sit at the kitchen table after Pa's call.

Am I overreacting?

This is the problem. You can know you're manic without necessarily being able to know whether or not the reactions you think are appropriate are out of proportion to the stimulus. It's hit or miss. Sometimes the awareness is there, sometimes not, and there's no knowing either way without hindsight and distance.

I envy how other people can go about interpreting the contents of their consciousness at face value, without question. The only recourse I have, I've found, is to approach the world with the belief that I am human first, Bipolar second, otherwise everything I ever experienced would be open to dispute and doing anything at all impossible.

Meditation and input from others might help if I suspect I'm overreacting when my climbing partner's called off or I've rowed with Aiyla, but with even a sniff of a threat of losing one of the handful of people you care for most in the world, there's not enough bandwidth left either side of the emotional maelstrom. This time, moreover, knowing that there's every chance that both Aiyla and Pa are only trying to talk me down for the sake of my sanity is enough to convince me that my instinct's on the nail.

It's a waiting game within the waiting game.

At dinner time there's a knock on my door. It's Giuseppina. She breaks into a wide grin when she sees me. She's holding a plate of bresaola. The bottoms of her rolled-up sleeves are dusted with flour.

'Your favourite!' she says, holding up the plate. 'I didn't see you today, so I wanted to bring you this and say thank you for the rent money you put—' Her smile retreats abruptly mid-sentence. 'Is something wrong?'

'Mia mamma,' I say, 'ha preso il virus.'

'Santo cielo, no!'

She places the plate down on my garden chair in the recess below the stairs and clasps her hands against her lips.

'No, Kieran. Don't cry, ti prego! Your mother is a strong woman. She will be fine.'

Through the blur of my own tears I see Giuseppina is crying too. I go to put a hand on her shoulder then remember I can't.

She listens wide-eyed, hands to her mouth, as I tell her what happened.

'We will pray for her this evening,' she says when I've finished. She takes the plate of bresaola from the chair and passes it to me, then points a finger towards the ceiling. 'I'm right here, remember, so don't you be alone. You have a family here. Worry about your mother but don't worry too much – it will do neither of you any good. And *eat*, I beg you.'

She blows me two kisses and returns upstairs.

I skip my nightly reading of *The Guardian*, CNN, and *Corriere della Sera*. The only news I care about is that which might arrive from a little semi-detached house on the east coast of Fife, Scotland.

Lockdown Day 47

I become a child again, bargaining with some imagined thunderer in the sky. I'll take another year of quarantine, never climb again, go home and settle down and be a better son, I tell Him, if only He'll let my mother be okay.

It's 3 a.m. I've been sitting watching Ma's WhatsApp profile for the past hour: 'Last seen yesterday at 21:09.'

She's had a hard life, Ma. Her brother died of leukaemia when he was three and Ma was six. Her first partner was abusive and hospitalised her on multiple occasions. When I was seven, a panic attack left her permanently blind in one eye and deprived her of her sense of taste and smell for almost fifteen years. For six years, after the death of her father, she looked after her sick mother seven days a week while working a full-time job, leaving home at six every morning and returning home at eight every night. Despite all this, she's the most incorrigibly cheerful, trusting, positive-minded and big-hearted person I've ever known. 'She's love personified,' Lucia told me after she and a group of friends from Valtellina had come to Scotland for a two-week climbing and hiking trip last summer. We'd planned on spending ten days in the Highlands but the group had become so fastened on Ma that we ended up leaving Fife a day late and returning two days early. She spent the time showing them how to bake scones, taking them to meet her friends, playing agony aunt at the kitchen table over endless cups of tea, feeding them up and sending them back to Italy with goody bags of homemade tablet, fudge and shortbread, and Lemsip.

The pain in my knee has worsened overnight and with every step there's a loud 'clack' that would suggest I'm going to need an operation sooner rather than later, but for now it seems an irrelevance. At 4 a.m. I set off on another hobbled sprint through the vineyard above town. I'm back by 5 a.m. and Ma's status on WhatsApp is the same. I do a few hours of work to distract myself, then some push-ups and sit-ups, all the while keeping my phone by my side. In a brief pause, I wonder how much of my hyperactivity can be ascribed to nervous energy and how much to mania, but have no way of knowing. The only thing I can be sure of is that staying still's not an option.

At 7.30 a.m. I hear Giuseppina in the garden and rush out to see her. She's crouching down on one knee at the front of the shed, watering a cluster of potted begonias she hasn't planted yet.

'Kieran, *caro*,' she says, 'what news do you have?'

'Nothing yet. I'm still waiting.'

'Go and sit down. I'll make us a coffee.'

Today I sit at the bottom of her stoop, my back against the

front wall beside the gate. Giuseppina turns her chair to face down the stairs.

'Don't torture yourself,' she says when I take my phone from my lap and check the screen for the dozenth time in the ten minutes we've been sat. 'She'll wake when she wakes. It's a good thing that she's sleeping.'

She hobbles down the stairs without me noticing. When I look up, she's reaching out a hand to pat my head.

Five minutes later, Ma's status changes to 'online'.

I hit the video-call toggle on my way down the stairs into the garden.

She's in bed, but sitting up.

'I'm okay,' she says when she answers. Her voice is a rattle, and her breath whinnying, but she looks brighter than yesterday. 'We just took my temperature and it's 38.3. That's not bad, I think.'

'How do you feel?'

'I think a bit better, but I'm not sure. My throat is awfully sore and I had a bit of bother breathing during the night, but I don't feel as hot or shivery.'

'Okay.'

Leaving her phone in her hand, she tilts her head back against the headboard. She's wearing a dressing gown. The collar on the t-shirt beneath it is loose where she's clawed around the neck to cool herself down.

'Today's your gran's birthday,' she says a few minutes later, the beginnings of a thin, stiff smile rising on her lips. 'She would have been ninety-six. It will be the first year I haven't been to the cemetery to see her.'

'Just stay in bed and rest, Ma. Don't think about anything else. I'm sure Gran would forgive you in the circumstances.'

I video-call again an hour later.

Pa appears on Ma's phone.

'She's sleeping,' he says. 'And maybe it's best we let her rest. Her phone's been going daft all day. Your aunty must have told the family. Anyway, she's exhausted. She's been that way for weeks but now this fever's just knocked her for six. We just have to be patient and hope. She has brighter moments, like this morning, but then—'

His voice tails off. A pair of tears race down his cheeks before he can lift a hand to cover his face.

I've never seen Pa cry before.

'Dad,' I say, as he angles the phone away, leaving me a view of the floor and the foot of the couch, where the dog's curled up at his slippered feet. 'Dad, it's okay.'

'I'm going to make her a cup of tea,' he says. 'I'll update you soon.'

I stammer through a few hours of work, then head to the Dusk Wall to keep myself busy and burn some of the nervous energy that's coursing through me. Someone is blaring opera again in the houses below. Verdi and Puccini, this time. There's an unmistakable lightness in the air that grates against my own mood. Is it just me?

I call Ma again before bed. Her temperature's still 38.2.

Lockdown Day 48

I wake early again and do a few hours of work while waiting for Ma to go online. When I step outside to get some fresh air, I find a white paper bag sitting on my doorstep. There's a Post-it attached to the front: *'Figurati! xxx'* ('You're welcome!')

Inside the bag I find a box of medication. My medication. It's a lower dose than I usually take but will be enough, I'm sure, to mitigate the stormiest of my internal weather for the time being. I'm too worried about Ma to celebrate, but quickly swallow the first of the new batch of thirty pills then text Holly to thank her.

She replies within a minute.

'Sorry it took so long! Got 'em on Tues but been knackered. Ur lights were off when I came up thru vines so didn't want to wake u. I'm going back to sleep now. U should 2! xxx.

'P.S. Volunteering for Red Cross now!'

It's only 5.20 a.m. I can't go back to sleep. Sleep would be a betrayal.

I'm in the kitchen. I can hear the mouse under my biscuit cupboard but he hasn't made an appearance yet.

I watch the clock on the wall above my kitchen table. The minute hand, I notice for the first time, is too thick, far too thick, taking up at least two increments instead of one. I take the clock down.

I call Ma as soon as I see she's awake.

She's smiling when she answers, but the lids of her eyes are so heavy that they hardly seem open.

'Listen to me,' she says. 'I can talk. And I'm not feeling nearly as fluey as I was. I'm not going to get excited because it's been coming and going, but it's definitely an improvement. Do I look better?'

She looks drained, her face pale and her eyes dark and ringed with purple, but the bluish tinge to her lips has gone and the wheezing from her lungs is less noticeable.

'You look great, Ma.'

She holds the phone to the side and coughs.

'I still have that, but I'm breathing better already.'

'Have you taken your temperature?'

'Your dad took it for me this morning. It's a bit lower – 38.1.'

'Okay.'

'Do you think that's okay?'

'I ... I don't know.'

'No, neither do we. When we were young you either had a temperature or you didn't. We didn't pay much attention to the specifics.'

'Wait.'

I google 'fever temperature'.

'Okay,' I say. 'Yesterday you had a high-grade fever, today you have a low-grade fever.'

'Well, that's good, isn't it?'

'Yeah, it must be. I still can't believe you can't see a doctor.'

'It's the Tories. They closed down all the surgeries.'

'Just promise me you'll go to the hospital if you feel it getting worse, okay? I know you want to be home but you'll get the best help there.'

'Okay, I promise.'

'And tell Dad to call or text me every hour with an update, okay?'

'Okay.'

I can't make sense of what's happened over the past few days. Weird as it was that Ma caught the virus in the first place, given how careful she's been, what's happened since then's been even weirder. She's had other symptoms for weeks, but the fever and shortness of breath usually last for as long as two weeks, from what I've gathered, whereas Ma's only had them for three days and already they appear to be easing off.

Around lunchtime I'm on my bed working when I hear the neighbour with the speakers playing 'Bella Ciao', the song of the *partigiani* who fought in the Italian Resistance against Mussolini and the Nazis during the Second World War. It's 25 April, the *Festa della Liberazione*, which commemorates the end of Nazi occupation. Over the past weeks, there has been much discussion about whether or not the usual parades and celebrations should be allowed, but thankfully the government has seen sense and decided to maintain lockdown. In the last week, the number of deaths has levelled off to around 450 per day, and allowing something like this, I'm sure, would only piss on all the hard work done thus far and lead to a resurgence in the numbers. Back home, a similar squabble has flared up over plans to celebrate our forebears' defeat of Nazism with a series of potentially self-destructive, contagion-conducive shindigs two weeks from now on VE Day, though the UK government's recent outage of logic and prudence inspires little faith that they'll follow the lead set by their Italian counterparts.

I try to catch up on the news to distract myself. My hand is shaking while I hold my phone and I have to steady it by clasping my wrist with the other. I open WhatsApp to check the dozen or so notifications I've received since last night. All of them are from Giuseppina's family and a former student of mine who knows the woman who found me at the gate two days ago, all of them sending their best wishes for Ma.

In the afternoon, Enzo comes to my door to ask if there's any news. I sit on the doorstep in my pyjamas and dressing gown. He stands across my terrace in his mask, backside against the railing.

'You have to remember that the 17 per cent death rate they're quoting for Lombardy is overstated because they've done so few tests on people not showing symptoms. That means it's a lot less lethal than we thought, so your mum's chance of surviving is huge. It's hard to think rationally or see things statistically in situations like this, I know, but try. Doing anything else is going to be agony.'

'Thank you, Enzo. You all doing okay?'

'Just waiting for the end. And it's not as if our *maldetto* government is helping. It's hard to believe anything they tell us because they change their minds all the time. It's like open-mic night in the bar and every arsehole in the country gets to pollute the air with whatever came to them in their dreams the night before. Conte has 450 advisers. Four hundred and fifty! What's that English saying? Too many cooks spoiling the broth? Here they're taking turns to piss in it and trying to feed it to us through our TVs every night. Then I see the pictures of those idiots protesting lockdown in the US and swarms of them going back to their beaches like the virus gives a shit that we're unhappy about our economies suffering and missing our summer. I know I should feel worried for them, but it just infuriates me. We have to work together. Doing it like this is like saying, Okay, we'll let some people shit in the pool but not the others. It doesn't work like that – if one place is swimming in shit, we all are. You know my father was a mountain guide, right? He always reminded me that you can only go as fast as the slowest member in your group. I have a feeling that member is going to be America. Imagine how much better the world would be if we had a mountain-goer in charge instead of these *deficienti* city people.'

Lockdown Day 49

I wake at 11 p.m.

I lie in bed trying to get back to sleep, but it doesn't happen. My hands are shaking and within a few minutes I notice I'm breathing like the clappers.

I move through to the living room and try to meditate, but I'm on my feet again within a minute. I go to the bathroom and pop a med, then pluck Aiyla's tube of lipstick from my counter and paint a huge pink graffito on my mirror: 'AND NOT TO YIELD'. I throw my clothes on, grab the rucksack that's been lying inside the door of my climbing cupboard since 7 March, almost fifty days ago, then sneak out the gate and down to my car.

I do my due diligence before starting the engine:

Are you manic?

Yes, most likely.

Are you doing something daft or dangerous?

Potentially, yes.

Is the need to do this daftness and/or dangerous thing justifiable (i.e. it will cause no harm to yourself or others) and are you doing it purely to reduce the risk of more serious daftness or danger later?

Yes.

Sure?

I turn the key in the ignition, kill the lights, then inch up the hill onto the Ponchiera road.

My heart's going apeshit, but a few hours from now, I know, it'll be worth it. It's a public service. Damage limitation. A different kind of 'appropriate safety measure'.

'Prevention's always better than cure,' I say aloud, then shush myself as I pass the last of the houses above the town.

Even before my auto-interrogation in the car, I knew my plan was solid and sound from all angles apart from a legal one. I'd drive up past the vineyards, through the little village of Ponchiera, and onto the back road for Valmalenco. I'd park before reaching Arquino in a little overgrown enclave beside a ruined house, then hike up through the forest to the crag at Valdone on the riverside footpath. I'd reach the crag around 1 a.m., climb until four, then roll the car back down the hill with the engine off and park up before anyone's awake.

It is, I think, fucking genius.

The Valdone crag is ideal: 100 or more metres of unpolished, blocky serpentine hidden in a wood at least 500 yards from the nearest road. I've considered the options subliminally over the past few weeks and landed here by a process of elimination: Sassella is too close to the road; Masso di Arquino is too small (if I'm going to break quarantine, the reward will have to justify the risk); and every other crag in the valley involves driving through town or on a busy road.

By the time I round the corner below Ponchiera, I'm bouncing in my seat, straining not to push the accelerator any harder and risk being heard by anyone in the houses either side of the road.

I've hit the straight between Ponchiera and Arquino when I see it – a light, that is, around half a mile in the distance. A house? Nah, it's moving.

Bollocks.

I slow down as the light approaches, hoping it will stop or divert.

It doesn't.

About 100 metres ahead of me there's a little wooded layby with benches overlooking the river at the bottom of the valley. I speed up, butt the car as deep as I can into the surrounding scrub, and kill the engine.

I duck my head and hold my breath as the car passes, then peer into the wing mirror to watch it receding into the distance and finally disappear.

Better to go home?

Yes.

Almost a quarter of a million people have died now globally. That's almost half the population of Edinburgh. Four full Hampden stadiums. I imagine that at least that many have felt the same cognitive dissonance as me in attempting to fathom how something we'd never heard of just a few months ago could be threatening to take away our loved ones while we sit by our phones, waiting on news, helpless to do more.

I call Ma at 8 a.m. UK time. Her temperature is down to 38.0. Her voice is crackly but less so than even yesterday.

'I've started to worry about your dad,' she says. 'He's been sleeping in our bed the last few nights instead of going into Cath's room, to keep an eye on me. We're sleeping top to tail to stay as far apart as possible, and we've got Rufus in between us, but that's the scariest thing about this blasted virus – we just don't know. And if he got it too, who'd take care of us?'

'Ma, now's not the time to be worrying about anything but getting yourself better. Just rest and try to relax. Put Dad on the phone.'

'What do you think is happening?' I ask Pa when he's taken

the phone into my sister's room and left Ma to go back to sleep. 'Most people who test positive have it for weeks, right?'

'I don't know. But she's not been right for ages: tired all the time, coughing. Maybe that was it and she's just been able to fight off the fever quicker. Would've helped if there'd been a doctor within a hundred miles, of course, but there isn't.'

'Are you feeling okay?'

'Aye. I got a bit of a fright the other day with your ma, obviously, but I've calmed down now that she's looking a bit better. I'm hoping that wee cough I had last week was as much as I'll see of it, but there's squat chance of getting tested. They opened that website for NHS staff and they were all booked up in minutes. The rest of us are just guessing. I'd feel a hell of a lot better if I could get in a climb or two somehow. Maybe I'll get along to the secret sea crag in St Monans if this good weather holds.'

'Dad . . .'

'Once your mum's better, obviously.'

Aiyla calls me later.

'I had therapy,' she tells me, after I've updated her on how Ma's doing and ask about her day.

'I know. Three sessions, right? Did they go okay?'

'No, I mean I *had* therapy, not gave therapy.'

'Oh.'

'Yeah, I know.'

'You didn't tell me.'

'I know. I didn't want to bother you with my stuff when all this is going on with your mum.'

'Bother me. Ma's getting better.'

'It's stupid.'

'If it made you feel you need help from a therapist, then it isn't stupid at all. Tell me what's been going on.'

'Lots of stuff, actually.'

'I have lots of time.'

'Being stuck here with my family's killing me – and we've only had five days of official lockdown. It's like you said. Everything is amplified, like you're seeing yourself under a microscope because you're finally staying still long enough to get a good look. You don't offload anything onto the world so the world's just offloading onto you. *Into* you. It's all input and no output, and all of the input's horrible. And then my clients. They all seem to be telling me exactly the same thing and it's fucking depressing.'

'What thing?'

'That the only way they can tolerate their lives and their circumstances is by living in a way that lets them escape those circumstances for a given number of hours every day. Now that they can't do that, they're crumbling.'

'Shit. Yeah, that is depressing.'

'What's even more depressing is that I'm starting to think it's true for almost everyone. I mean, isn't it?'

'Maybe. But that can be a good thing, right?'

'How?'

'Imagine there was a silver lining – that, despite being undoubtedly the shittest thing to happen in our lifetimes, this whole tragedy turned out to be a turning point and the launchpad to the things our planet and species have been crying out for for years.'

'Honey, hundreds of thousands of people have died.'

'I know. But the fallout from all those deaths and all this

suffering could be the catalyst for the kind of change that was impossible to even dream of before this all kicked off. Before any of this happened, we were just drifting along, accepting the unacceptable by virtue of its familiarity and because our unhappiness, stress, discontent and the levels of ugliness and shittiness always registered just below the critical mass required to mobilise people, to trigger the need to make change. Without this, we might have gone on doing it all our lives. Now, people have got to be waking up. And in the same way as the virus might be the launchpad for changing the people we put into power, how we treat each other, how we treat the planet, it might also be the launchpad for changing how we live our lives. You're right, we've been forced to look at things like we normally never do. You know Rumi, right? He said, "These pains you feel are messengers; listen to them." Well, people are listening now and—'

'Slow down!' she barks. 'Why are you talking so fast?'

Am I talking fast?

After our call, I try to replay our conversation in my head, but can't remember any more than the last few exchanges. I think about calling back or sending a voice message, but know my internal censor will slow me down to compensate. Instead, I try out a few lines in front of the mirror.

'There'sachanceImightbetalkingfastbutIcan'tbesurebecause therearenospeedometersforspeechandevenifIwastalkingfast-maybemybrainwouldbeworkingtoofastforthefastnesstoregister.'

Was that fast?

I don't know. My lips were moving – the way people's lips move when they speak.

Really?

Okay. Maybe a bit fast.

Keep an eye on it?

Yeah.

Giuseppina comes to my door around lunchtime to ask about Ma. She's brought me another plate of bresaola.

'I wanted to hear about your mother,' she says, handing me the plate, 'and make sure you're eating.'

'She's much better. It's like a miracle. They told her older people can have delayed presentation of fever and respiratory symptoms, which seems to be what happened to her. But they seem to be going away already. It's only been five days.'

'Didn't I tell you there was no use in worrying?' she says, clasping her hands in front of her face.

I want to hug her but as she gazes up at me I can see that she's already hugging me with her eyes.

'She's not in the clear yet,' I say, 'but she's getting there.'

'Of course. It will take time. But now you must let yourself relax a little bit. She will be okay. I can feel it. I remember the last time Domenico went into hospital. I despaired when they took him away in the ambulance because I knew that time he wouldn't be coming back, even though he'd been in a dozen times before and I'd thought no such thing. I'm no mystic, but we all have ways of knowing these things, don't you think?'

Lockdown Day 50

Day 50.

I'm high when I wake. Unmistakably. Unbecomingly, given that my mother's still in the throes of a battle with a life-threatening virus.

I'm hoping this is just a hangover, a withdrawal symptom from the few weeks when I was rationing my meds, and that the pills Holly sourced from her doctor friend will kick in soon and level things off.

It's not the first time that the clash between circumstances and my neurocircuitry has led to inappropriate behaviour. In the past, I've had to skip funerals and christenings to avoid causing a scene. I lost my university girlfriend when I started reciting poetry to her father in a crowded restaurant in a bid to console him for the death of his mother a fortnight previously. In the week after 9/11, I was arrested in Arizona for riding a kids' tricycle through the streets of Tempe, Phoenix, in the early hours of the morning while singing, the report stated, 'Ob-la-di, Ob-la-da' at the top of my voice and then attempting to embrace the officer who'd pulled me over. He wasn't a hugger.

I call Ma as soon as she's awake.

'37.5!' she says, before I can say hello. She disappears from the screen for a moment to cough. The cough is coarse but less violent than it has been, and when she returns her face is ruddier and eyes brighter than they have been in weeks.

'I had a good sleep last night,' she says, 'and I wasn't feeling that same shivery or sweaty way that I have been. I'm just praying it continues.'

'It will, Ma. Just keep resting up. You aren't out of the woods yet.'

'Just as well you never tried to become a motivational speaker.'

'You know what I mean.'

'Yes. Now just you get on with your work and don't worry about me. Your dad's taking good care of me. He's been a star. It's been hard for him, not being able to climb and now probably wondering if he's going to get this himself. But he's been up and down the stairs every half-hour to check up on me and bringing me cups of tea. Maybe I should get one of these viruses more often, eh?'

'Ma . . .'

'Yes, you're right. Still a little too soon . . .?'

It rained heavily overnight, but when I check on the azalea the ground doesn't seem waterlogged and the plant looks healthy despite my neglect over the last few days. The pointed buds are no bigger than almonds, but some have already started to open, revealing the pale lips of the petals and emanating a fresh, perfumy scent that reminds me of my grandmother.

I've already put in six hours' work by noon so I decide to take an early lunchbreak and get in a few traverses on the Scorpion Wall. Between climbs, I see more people walking on Via Scarpatetti than I have done since the beginning of quarantine and can't be sure if I'm encouraged.

After climbing, I go inside to check the news. 'Now Is the Time to Coexist with the Virus,' reads the headline in *Il Giorno*, quoting Prime Minister Giuseppe Conte. Last night, I missed his announcement outlining the plans for Phase 2, moving the country out of lockdown. I find a video on *La Repubblica* but it's almost an hour long and after ten minutes of watching Conte's drained, fumbling explanation of what's coming next, I scroll down to a link to the new, updated *decreto*, only to find seventy pages of convoluted legalese from which I glean only a few crumbs of intelligible information.

Here's what I gather:

From 4 May we'll be able to visit relatives as long as there are no gatherings or parties. The travel ban between regions remains, but we can travel within our own *comune*. Public parks will be reopened and outdoor exercise will be allowed within them, without restrictions or police checks, as long as there's compliance with social distancing. Hugs and hand-shakes are discouraged. Restaurants will be open for takeaways but not sit-in dining. Funerals can be held with a maximum of fifteen socially-distanced mourners. The price of masks, which will be mandatory in all public spaces, will be fixed at 0.50 cents. Shops and cultural sites will reopen on 18 May. Bars, restaurants and hairdressers on 1 June. There's no mention of climbing or mountaineering.

Do national parks count as public parks?

I phone my climbing partner, Matteo, for clarification. As much as the pills from Holly will help, I know I won't be out of the woods until I'm back to getting my daily fill of normal exercise and fresh air. From experience, I know that every day without an outlet for the surfeit of energy building up inside of me is usually another in the direction of calamity.

'So, are we allowed to go climbing or not?' I ask him.

'It wasn't very clear. Instead of Phase 2, it's more like a Phase 1.5. I didn't get it either. I've been online, checking in the climbing chat groups, but nobody knows. Or rather, everybody thinks they know something different from the other. Even people who've read the whole *decreto* say there are around a dozen points that suggest yes and a dozen that suggest no. Wait ... Here it is: "*Movement is allowed for proven professional needs, health reasons or necessity.*" And then: "*It is not permitted to take part, in the outdoors, in activities that are recreational or ludic.*" I looked up "ludic" a few minutes ago and apparently it means, basically, "fun". And this was one of the clear parts. Who knows what the fuck the rest of it means.'

'So it's a "no", then?'

'It looks like it. Unless you happen to have an ibex or mountain goat for a mother-in-law or are burying someone in a rock face. But some of the papers are saying we can go to the mountains as long as we stay two metres apart and don't drive to get there. Then some of them say we need an *autocertificazione*, which would mean "no" because you have to declare that you can prove you're going somewhere for work or health reasons.'

'So a "maybe"?'

'Yeah. But there are still seven days to go. Don't bet against them changing everything before we get there.'

At dinner time I'm still full of energy, despite having woken at 3.30 a.m. and put in my daily quota of climbs on my lunch-break. The clouds that blanketed the valley this morning have dispersed and the sun has dried the worst of last night's rainfall, so I head up to the Dusk Wall.

I hear voices from different directions and see more people strolling up and down Via Scarpatetti, around five in the first twenty minutes of climbing – it seems that the announcement of the new *decreto* has been to some townspeople what the dinner bell was to the salivary glands of the Pavlovian dog.

The stone is still slightly damp but its coarseness on my skin and the movement of my muscles feels like salve on a wound. The crickets are out, their shrill song like that of a thousand tiny bugles announcing the arrival of summer. The burnt scent of the rock triggers a mental collage of imagery from past climbs, transporting me to airy spots high on the walls of Val di Mello, Glen Etive, The Trapps in upstate New York, Cima Grande di Lavaredo in the Dolomites, Shepherd's Crag in Borrowdale. The memories are bittersweet, evoking a feeling that rests somewhere between longing and comfort. The more I indulge them, however, the more I'm inclined to question how much longer the garden's blessed but modest walls can help keep me on the safe side of unhinged and stave off an episode. While the outlet they've provided me all this time has been priceless, I feel like I'm playing catch-up, trying to slough with a spoon a burden of surplus hyperthymic voltage replenished daily by the bucketful.

I need out. I'm trying to convince myself I'm doing okay but the effort's stealing the strength I need to keep okay on the cards for much longer. Meds aren't enough. Video chats aren't enough. Meditation isn't enough. I need to climb.

While I'm climbing, though, a strange feeling creeps up on me, one that's inexplicable, kinda nauseating, and impossible to square with the urgency of my need to re-establish my routines: *I'm scared about the end of the quarantine.* I've become used to the serenity, the silence, the certainty of what each day will look like. I try to imagine the day when the quarantine's over, when we walk out of our homes and into the world on the other side of 3 May, but the vision stalls somewhere between my front door and the gate. The idea of that kind of freedom suddenly feels, inexplicably, overwhelming.

The highest peak I've ever climbed was only some 6,200 metres – a modest peak in Himalayan terms, but around double the height at which most people begin to experience altitude sickness. Climbing a peak of that height, the process of altitude acclimatisation can take days, maybe weeks, depending on the reaction of the individual. I have a feeling that, for most of us, it will be the same with the reopening, with the freedom that awaits us once restrictions are loosened. Just as we were new-comers to the quarantine experience, we'll be newcomers to the experience of whatever awaits us on the other side of quar-antine, which is sure to be every bit as disorienting and just as much, if not more, of a culture shock. The re-acclimatisation will be piecemeal and halting, not just on a national level, I'm sure, but individually. Though I'd like to think I'll be able to hit the ground running, pick up where I left off and start making up for lost time with a month-long odyssey of all the climbs I was dreaming of until just a few days ago, the nearer we get to reopening, the less I'm able to imagine it. Just the thought of rushing out on day one of post-quarantine gives me a nosebleed. Is it the risk of infection I'm scared of, or the freedom?

Lockdown Day 51

My newsfeed on Facebook is awash with conflicting interpre-tations on the government's *decreto*, most of them concerned with the vagueness or lack of explicit reference to visiting the mountains and climbing. The lowest common denominators of the hive brain have concluded that we a) have free rein to do whatever we wish and have the document's vagueness as our defence, or b) can do nothing and, therefore, should revolt and do whatever the hell we want regardless. The more rational and typo-, expletive- and emoji-free observations agree that we can go anywhere we wish as long as we respect rules on social distancing and do so under our own steam, i.e. either on foot or by bicycle.

'Looks like we're almost out of it,' I tell Giuseppina over our morning coffee.

She looks uncharacteristically listless, gazing thoughtfully over the garden with her lips pursed in a pout.

'So they tell me.' She sips from her cup, then glances back over the railing and shrugs with an unreadable smile.

'You don't look so pleased.'

'It doesn't make much difference to me. I want my children and grandchildren to enjoy their lives and go on their travels and to university and so on, but I've enjoyed having everyone around. This,' she waves her arm around her, 'this is my world. I only know what comes into it. The presidents, the mayors, and those terrors in England and America and Brazil – none of that means much to me. I only hope that what they do does no harm to my family and they can come to visit me so I can see they are happy and well. That's all. And you've been here more too, of course. It's been nice to have you, even if I know you're missing your mountains. I see it in your eyes, you know.'

'I just don't know if it's a good thing, the reopening,' I say. 'It feels too soon.'

'My grandfather, who lived in the house I showed you on Via Scarpatetti before the wars, told us a story when we were children, about a farmer. The farmer had only one horse and one day the horse escaped from his paddock. The farmer's neighbours all came to console him and said, "Oh, that's terrible!", but the farmer smiled and said, *"Vedremo"* [We'll see]. Then, a few weeks later, the farmer's horse returned with another horse, a mate, so now the farmer had two horses. The neighbours came and said, "How fortunate!", but the farmer only smiled and said, *"Vedremo."* A few weeks later, the farmer's son was trying to break in the new horse but it threw him off and the boy broke his hip. When the farmer told his neighbours, they all said, "What bad luck!", and again the farmer only replied, *"Vedremo."* Another few weeks passed, then an army arrived in the farmer's village, conscripting all the able young men to go to war, but because the farmer's son was still unable to walk, he was excused and left behind.'

She grins down at me between the bars of the banister.

'I forget the rest of it, but you get the point.'

I put in twelve hours of work trying to make up for all I've missed over the past few days. According to the reports I've been reading on the impact of social-distancing measures on airline ticket prices, the money I'd earmarked first for Patagonia and then flights for my post-quarantine hugging spree might only be enough to fund a visit home when they finally reopen the borders.

I call Ma every few hours. Her temperature is down to 37.2 and she's breathing normally.

In the evening I go to the Dusk Wall before sunset. Though in the shadow of the castle hill, the rock is still warm. Lizards have posted themselves like fidgety sentinels at two-foot intervals, warming their bellies on my holds.

I'm still jittery. Though I've tried to meditate for the past few days, each time I've only managed ten or fifteen minutes before losing concentration and giving up: as with the stay-at-home order, I'm finding that the more I need to do something, the harder it is to do it. At the end of the first traverse I close my eyes and try to do the climb in reverse by feel alone. On the first attempt, I have to cheat by opening my eyes to locate holds I can't remember, but by the fifth try I manage to go end-to-end without having to pause for more than a few seconds before any move. There's a childishness to it, of course, but the shutting-down of one of the senses focuses and heightens the attention of the others, turning the process into a form of moving meditation. A few moves in, everything seems new: the sweet mustiness of the cooling grass and acrid scent of the rocks; the crusty, dimpled surface of each hold beneath my fingertips; the pressure of my weight on my toes; the flexing of my joints.

By the end of the first traverse my attention is stable, no longer flighty and flitting. The quietening of the permachatter in my brain and clearing of the grainy fug that descends over it during long days at my computer makes it feel like Reality 2.0, highlighting the gulf between this and the fuzzy, automaton daze with which I go about the rest of my days. For almost a week, my heartbeat has been irregular and skittish – nothing out of the ordinary but symptomatic of the anxiety and tension concurrent with most episodes of mania, no matter how mild. Now, I feel it decline in real time to a steady, metronomic rhythm and a general ease suffuses my body as a whole.

I hear my neighbour Attilio's goat baying. He's at the fence, watching me through the trees. I scoot down the hill to feed him some grass and see my neighbour Fausto on the far side of Attilio's garden, about 40 metres away, but no sign of Attilio. Fausto starts making his way across the sloping plot when he sees me. On the way he passes the kid, Teresina, and scoops her into his arms.

'Look at this little delight,' he says as he approaches, his thin, grainy voice barely audible over the rustling of the trees in the warm wind blowing up the valley from the west.

'She's growing fast,' I say.

He plants a kiss on Teresina's head, then puts her down on the grass.

I see that Teresa, her mother, is tied up.

'Has she been out without the *autocertificazione*?' I ask.

'No, this was Attilio's choice. He's gone up to visit his boys for a few days. They're up there,' he says, pointing across the valley towards Pizzo Meriggio, which still wears a thick, bright cap of snow on the last 300 metres or so below the peak, 'in their *baita* on the mountain. He sent them there two months ago for safety, and they haven't been down since. He asked me to look after the animals while he's visiting them and making sure they're keeping up with their schoolwork, not destroying the place. Where have you been the past few days? I haven't seen you.'

I tell him about Ma.

'Caspita' (Good heavens), he says. 'Just as well she's a young-ster. What is she, fifty?'

'Sixty-nine.'

'Ah, *beh*. A youth. She will be fine, I'm sure. And you, are you well?'

'I'll be a lot better when they let us out and we can start putting all of this behind us.'

'The end is a long way off yet, *ragazzo*. We can't grasp it at the moment because we're still inside it, but I believe that when my grandchildren and their children study all this ten, twenty, fifty years from now, this – what we've been through – will be like the bullet that hit the archduke, noth-ing more. The rest of it is yet to come. And when they try to understand it, they'll see that the bullet was inevitable, that the hallmarks of what we've experienced these past months, and which allowed this horror to occur, are the result of things put in motion years and years ago.'

Fausto pauses to wave to the two Marias – Maria Rosa and Maria Grazia, who've been doing laps of Via Scarpatetti and the staircase all afternoon and are now passing below his vegetable plot – then resumes, raising one of his bony, scarred fingers to ensure my attention hasn't drifted to Teresina, who's broken into an impromptu mosh on the slope between the pear trees behind him.

'My only hope,' he continues, 'is that all this horror has forced enough people to look. You have to look at something before you can see it is sick. Take my plants – if I see one of them has a disease or aphids, then I treat it. It would be easier, of course, to leave it be and carry on with my other business, but if I don't, eventually they die. Simple. Italy is sick. The world is sick.'

Lockdown Day 53

Holly texts in the morning asking if I can help with her shopping. She wants to stock up so she can avoid going back to the supermarket again soon but is still too weak to carry everything alone.

I meet her by the fountain in Piazza Quadrivio, outside Vittorio's store. When I see her through the final archway at the bottom of Via Scarpatetti, I hardly recognise her. Her yellow puffer jacket hangs off her like a small poncho. When she sees me coming, she grins. Her teeth are grotesquely large in her withered face.

She pulls her mask up over her nose and mouth.

'Don't worry,' she says. 'I'm sure I'm not infectious any more, but just to be safe ...'

The transformation is even more startling up close. Almost half of her is missing.

She leans back and props herself up on the rim of the fountain behind her.

'It's so good to see you,' she says, giving me a wave in lieu of *baci*. Her soft, earthy Manchester drawl is medicinal, a kindly dose of a normality preceding even the one that existed before quarantine.

'You, too,' I say. 'What's left of you.'

'Ah, yeah,' she shrugs. 'Covid diet.'

'I didn't expect to hear from you. I thought you'd be busy with the Red Cross.'

'I had to quit. Long story.'

It is.

Vittorio's store is closed for Labour Day so we go to the supermarket in the town centre. On the way, and for another three or four hours after we've fetched her groceries, she barely pauses for breath while updating me on everything that's happened since we last spoke and filling in all the blanks from around and before the time she started showing symptoms.

She starts at the beginning.

She went home for Christmas in the UK. Her family met to have dinner together and by the time she returned to Italy in early January, seven of the twelve family members at the dinner had fallen ill with some form of throat infection and cough. Throughout January and February, Holly had an intermittent cough and at the beginning of March developed the fever that she's had on and off ever since. When she went to visit her doctor, she was told to rest up and take aspirin for seven days. After four days, her temperature was a full two degrees above her regular one and the cough had 'started to sound like a bloomin' death rattle'. She returned to the doctor, who by now had a hacking cough of his own. By this point, the Italian association of medical professionals had issued guidelines on diagnosis to doctors around the country. Before being given a test for Covid-19 and admitted to hospital, patients had to have a temperature of 37.8 and be showing symptoms of a fever, cough and respiratory problems.

'The trouble was,' Holly says, 'my normal temperature is 35.5 Celsius, so when I told my doctor my thermometer was reading 37.3 and his confirmed it, he thought I was being paranoid and told me just that. "Go home and rest up. You'll be fine," he said.'

Her apartment building is in the *cittavecchia*, hidden in the labyrinth of tiny, crooked cobbled streets behind the church, all of which barely get started before ending or veering off at oblique angles into further concealed passageways. We climb the narrow stairwell to her apartment on the first floor and drop off her groceries. While we're laying the bags inside the entrance, I notice she's out of breath and for maybe the fifth time already that morning wonder if she might still be conta- gious. I pull my mask tighter over my nose. After leaving her groceries, we climb another flight of stairs, first to a narrow landing above the courtyard, then through a tunnel-like cor- ridor lined with bicycles that leads into the garden.

'So,' she says, pulling out a pair of mildewed garden chairs from behind a tree near the back of the overgrown lawn, 'I went home and rested up and, lo and behold, my fever popped up to 37.5 and my lungs started to feel more and more like a furnace, so I phoned the doctor for another appointment. This time, he was a little more sheepish and accepted that maybe I had something. Either, he said, bronchitis, pneumonia or Covid. We ruled out bronchitis because the symptoms I had were too severe. Then he listened to my lungs and ruled out pneumonia. "Okay," I thought, "we're making progress." But then he put his stethoscope away and sat back down behind his desk and told me, "*Signora*, you're a healthy young lady. You have a cough and a bad throat, but I have a cough and a bad throat. Do you see anyone taking me into the Covid ward? No. Your temperature is normal. You don't have Covid. Go home, rest, take aspirin. You'll be fine in a few days." So, I went home, took my aspirin and went to bed. The next morning my temperature was up to 37.7 and I was starting to panic. I tried calling him but it was a Saturday and he wasn't answering. So, I spoke to my doctor friend, Francesco, who lives in the next building. He diagnosed me from his window, 10 metres away, with all the neighbours listening in from their balconies. He'd already treated patients with Covid so it only took him two minutes to tell me what that silly twat – excuse my French – couldn't tell me in two weeks and that I should call an ambulance.

'When the Red Cross people came, they took my oxygen levels. They were at 91 per cent – 1 per cent higher than the figure for automatic hospitalisation. They gave me the choice of going to the Covid ward for critical patients at Morelli, which is about 20 bloody miles away, or staying here, so I decided to stay. It was daft, I know, but I reasoned that people who go into Morelli don't come out – not alive, anyway – so

for the next week Francesco suited up in his hazmat and ferried me back and forward from the hospital for tests on my
lungs, heart and blood, and got me started on the high dosage
of vitamin C. It was touch and go for a while. I was shitting it.
I called my brother and got him to put a digital signature on
my will and told him where to scatter my bloody ashes – half
of them along the banks of the Adda at Parco Bartesaghi and
half on Durness beach, in case you're wondering. Anyway,
I have no doubt that I wouldn't be here telling you this if
Francesco hadn't been there and got me started on the vitamin
C treatments and convinced me to call the ambulance. I nearly
died, all because that man was too stubborn to consider that
his diagnostic tools might be off.'

I realise this is the first chance she's had to speak English in
over two months. Her phone's rung at least four times since
we sat down and she hasn't even looked to see who's calling.

'But, to be fair to him, it's all dead messy. Half of the people
in the Covid hospital in Sondalo have tested negative, despite
the fact that it's exclusively for the most extreme cases. Some
of them have tested negative with oxygen levels as low as 40
per cent. They're swabbing people's nasal cavities and throats
when the bloody virus has already migrated to their lungs.
The swabs are only useful in the early stages. And one of
my friends died whose only symptom for the first weeks was
conjunctiv-bloody-itis.'

'But you were better when I spoke to you. I thought you'd
made a full recovery.'

Her neighbours are cooking in their garden, a similarly
sized rectangle to Holly's on the tier below. The scent of
real food after subsisting on a supermarket-avoidance diet of

canned sweetcorn, chickpeas and tuna for the past two months has me salivating in my seat.

'I had,' she says, 'kinda. For about a week, I only had a cough and a sore throat. That's when we spoke on the phone. When I started getting my strength back, I managed to sign up for the Red Cross on the day they reopened – by then they were so desperate that they were accepting anyone daft enough to volunteer. I just wanted to do something and they needed ambulance drivers and helpers to distribute masks. Back at the start of it all, I petitioned the MP in my constituency back home and wrote up a few advisories for people who weren't in lockdown yet and they've all gone viral on social media. But I wanted to do more *here*. Then, I was sitting at home making all these masks I planned on distributing to whoever needed them, and I realised my symptoms were coming back. I was in bed for another two weeks, sweating, not sleeping, eating like a sparrow – hence the new, lithesome version of Holly you see before you now. I was gutted, but I managed to keep things going even when I was sick. I joined a class action group that's building a court case for people who've been misdiagnosed or lost family because of mistakes made by their doctors or employers and I've been trying to help the kids in Brescia and Bergamo orphaned by the virus. I trained as a psychologist before I became a teacher, so I've been doing trauma counselling with the older kids when I can.'

'I've been climbing the walls in my garden and planting flowers. The sum total of my altruism amounts to a few biscuit crumbs I've been leaving out for the mouse in my kitchen.'

'Ah, you do what you can do, right? Besides, mice and flowers need love as much as humans do, eh?'

'I'd give you a hug and a pat on the back if I thought there wasn't a chance it might kill me. Which reminds me, why are you stocking up on food if you've already had it? I mean, if we're supposing having antibodies gives you immunity.'

'Oh, mate,' she says, tilting her head with a wry smile. 'Peeps in South Korea are already getting a second bout and I'm not gonna be ready for round two for a lonnnnng time.'

One of her neighbours calls up from the garden below.

We head back down the stairs, where, beneath an arbour smothered in ivy, four of her neighbours are sitting at a stone table in front of a huge plate of polenta, a platter of grilled pork ribs and a bowl of tossed salad. One of the neighbours shuffles over on his seat to make room for Holly when he sees us coming, leaving a space that, even given her new, diminished proportions, will place them no more than a foot apart when she sits.

'Wait,' I say, 'are you all going to eat together?'

'Yeah, this is the Covid Café, matey. We've all had it. We're doing our bit for herd immunity in this *palazzo*. Boris would be proud.'

Lockdown Day 54

I get a call from Lucia's brother, Michele, at 6.30 a.m.

'*Ueilà,*' he says when I answer.

'It's 6.30 a.m.,' I say.

'*Si, si,*' he says, 'almost lunchtime.'

My friendship with Michele began upon his discovery that I was one of few others in the valley who shared his affinity for the early hours of the morning and was thus available to keep him company on the epically long ski-mountaineering days for which he sets off not long after most people are going to bed.

He's right. I've been awake for hours, trying to work but getting nowhere. My brain appears to be protesting against the overload of stimuli and stress it's been assaulted with this past week and has chosen to boycott anything more taxing than browsing the news and watering Giuseppina's plants.

'I thought you said things couldn't get any worse after Trump and Brexit, eh?'

'I'm still not sure the first one's gonna be less deadly than the virus. How's Simona?'

'Lucky she works in a hospital in Switzerland and not Italy. Here they send nurses to war with feathers and prayers, there they send them with tanks. She went back to our apartment the day this all kicked off. I was at my parents' place looking after my mum and got trapped, so I haven't been able to see her since then, but I'm hoping they'll let me go back on Monday – we have the *affetti stabili* [stable affections] they mentioned being necessary for home visits in the latest *decreto*, after all. If that's the marker, though, I reckon half the husbands and wives in the country will be out on the street by then. You doing okay?'

'Yeah. It's been rough, but we're nearly there. Reopening's just three days away.'

'Reopening my arse. They've left a gap in the door, nothing more. Not yet. And I have no faith that this four-week, staged reopening's gonna go smoothly. Anyway, I have some serious business to discuss with you,' he says, his voice turning that droll way I'm used to hearing when he's about to suggest we ski up and down something in an afternoon that most people would do over two days. 'Do you want a job?'

'I have one.'

'A real job, I mean. Sitting on your arse at your computer scribbling shit all day doesn't count, not in Valtellina.'

Michele's a gamekeeper and wildlife-management special-ist, and spends months at a time living out of his tent and huts in Stelvio National Park, the Orobie and the Rhaetic Alps. He sends me photos almost daily to remind me of his good fortune, usually when he knows I'm particularly under the cosh and stuck in the house at my computer.

'Ah, you mean shooting defenceless critters up in the mountains?'

'No, dickhead. I mean in the vineyard. I managed to sneak Lucia back over the border a few days early by putting her on the books as an employee, and—'

'Lucia's back?'

'Yeah. Vineyards are considered an "essential" business. I've been working solid these past two months and I needed someone to help me out. My dad's out of action. He had a little accident on the tractor and broke his arm, so I've been on my own. Lucia's been a big help, but it would be handy to have someone who's not averse to the heavy work. With Dad out of commission, I thought I'd headhunt the next biggest, smartest, hardest-working guy in the valley. Is my flattery working?'

'I'll need to check my schedule.'

'Fuck your schedule. Sleep's for resort skiers and Milanese, remember? I'll give you a call next week. I'll see if I can't maybe wangle something to get Matteo and Simona here, too.'

Ninety hours from now, the door that was slammed shut fifty-three days ago (fifty-seven, by then) will be partially reopened, and neither the reopeners nor those behind the door have the slightest clue what to expect or, despite the zealousness of their cries of yay or nay, whether it's the right move.

'We're on the way down,' Michele told me earlier. 'And every mountaineer knows what happens on the way down . . .'

Roughly 80 per cent of mountaineering accidents occur on the descent. We relax, thinking the hard work's done, and let complacency sneak in, despite being on the same mountain, the same distance above a hard landing, exposed to just the same dangers as we were on the way up – just as I learned to my expense on that afternoon on Corno Stella four years ago. Being 500 metres from the ground on the way up, alas, is the same as being 500 metres from the ground on the way down, just as having 50,000 infected people on the upward curve is the same as having 50,000 infected people on a downward one. The consequences of negligence are the same, the responsibilities to our *compagni di cordata* ('rope partners') no less exigent.

Since the announcement and publication of the latest *decreto,* the shift in mindset has been apparent, and done little to inspire anything like faith in a smooth, hitch-free return to better times. Every day this past week, I've seen around twenty, mainly unmasked, non-resident walkers on Via Scarpatetti, an increase of around nineteen on the average for the five previous weeks. Elisa and Enzo tell me that when they've been making their way to and from work in the town centre, it's been as though the townspeople equate the forthcoming easing of restrictions with the virus's demise, with most people they pass flouting distancing rules, unmasked and casually socialising *al fresco* wherever they can – outside newsagents, on benches, in any of the countless little alleys that branch off from the main arteries of the town centre. Pictures from Milan, Rome and Pavia in the newspapers in the past few days have shown a larger-scale version of the same. Consorting is the new contraband.

Lockdown Day 55

Bad news: travelling by car to other *comune* is still prohibited, meaning climbing is still off the cards for now. Sondrio used to have a crag on the cliffs below the Chiesa di San Bartolomeo, the sixteenth-century church that stands on a rocky bluff above the River Mallero. In my first year here, I'd gone to check it out one afternoon, only to be chased away by an angry priest while I was setting up an abseil to do some recce on the rock face below. Now, the nearest crag is in Sassella.

They're calling it a 'false reopening'. While we're allowed to leave our homes, little else has changed. Again, the differences in response of my country of birth and my adoptive one are telling. In the UK, four in five people don't think it's time to reopen; here people are preparing to riot because the loosening of restrictions has undone only a few of the stitches instead of ripping open the seams.

I receive a text from Luigi, asking if I want to climb on Monday. I spent the morning scouring Facebook and every Italian climbing and mountaineering blog I know in search of a more favourable interpretation of the *decreto* and in particular the part about travel to another *comune*. At some point, I realised that I was wasting my time, that it doesn't matter whether the *decreto* allows us to travel to other *comuni* or not. Even if it were permitted, would I go, and risk bringing the virus back here, to Giuseppina? Supposing just ten people had climbed the same routes we chose to climb before us, that's ten chances of infection. And if either Luigi or I had it, then having to share our equipment would make us highly susceptible to passing it on to each other over the course of a two- or three-hour session.

'*We could wear masks and gloves?*' writes someone in our WhatsApp climbing group.

'*Why don't we just wear our harnesses round our necks and fill our chalk bags with lube instead?*' someone else replies.

It seems solo climbing might be the only way. In summers past, I've often gone to crags at 4 or 5 a.m. to climb before temperatures get too high and learned to lead-solo* at least a few routes at each crag so I'd be able to climb alone if, as was usually the case, I couldn't find anyone else disposed to such an early start. But before doing that again, I want to see which Italy turns up in the reopening: the unofficial one or the official one; the Italy that follows an unwritten '70 means 90' rule regarding traffic speed limits and is releasing Mafia members by the dozen from prison, or the one that writes up seventy-page lists of instructions for lockdown, imposes prob-ably the strictest quarantine in the world, and fills the prison spaces vacated by those *mafiosi* with people caught jogging alone in the forests and vineyards.

My assignments for the first half of May arrived in my inbox during the night. I still have two remaining from April for

---

* Climbing with a rope, but without a partner, using a self-belay device for safety.

which I've been given an extension, but it looks like I'll be spending a lot more of my post-quarantine freedom than I'd like stuck in front of my computer trying to make up for my laxness over the past few weeks and my brain's refusal to cooperate over the last three or four days.

I sit down at my computer at 4 a.m. to make a start, but it's the same as yesterday and the day before. At 6.30 a.m. I'm still in my seat, on my third coffee, and have done no more than write the title to my penultimate post for April. This has happened before, but usually I manage to get something approaching readable onto the page by dint of perseverance. Today: nothing.

At 8 a.m. I put in ten traverses on the Dusk Wall and another five on Indecent Exposure. After coffee with Giuseppina, I return to my computer and squeeze out a paragraph that barely qualifies as English.

I try again throughout the day, hoping some inspiration will miraculously appear, but it doesn't happen.

I go back to the Dusk Wall before dinner to put in another few traverses. Afterwards, I'm marvelling at the deep-green tones of the forests on the other side of the valley, which only a few weeks ago were still garbed in their tawny winter plumage, when something interrupts me. I look up and see Giuseppina on the small, square balcony outside her kitchen, hanging out tea towels to dry in the warm evening breeze.

'Who are you talking to, *caro*?' she asks, her frown offset by a slant of humour in her eyes.

Had I been talking to myself? My recollection of the past few minutes is almost nil, but a backwards glance into the contrails of my racing thoughts turns up a few incoherent mutterings about azaleas and something to do with cigars.

Luckily, I have my headphones in from the call I'd made to Ma while doing my traverses. I pluck one from my ear and wave it above my head.

'Ah, thank goodness!' Giuseppina says. 'I thought I was going to have to call the *manicomio* and lose my helper.'

Her laugh is interrupted by a second thought.

'Excuse me, Kieran,' she says, her face straightening. 'Of course, I didn't mean any offence.'

Shit.

I phone Aiyla when I get back inside.

Over the years, my Bipolar's become like a vetting mechanism whenever I meet new people, their reactions when I 'come out' giving me ample forewarning as to whether or not they'll turn out to be sympathetic to the condition. The reactions to date have ranged from soul-crushing to hilarious – from ghosting before ghosting was a thing to the marginally more common, 'Oh, we're all a bit like that, aren't we?' None of them, alas, have encouraged or emboldened me to share more frequently or freely in future.

I told Aiyla early on in our relationship. I wanted to give her the chance to back off; to save us both disappointment; to avoid potential claims of false advertising somewhere down the line. But I also tried to downplay the condition as much as possible – a policy I've always been aware I might one day live to regret. At the start, I was able to rationalise making light of things with a number of justifications that seemed reasonable at the time: because I was already scared of scaring her off and losing her; because I didn't want my condition to be the thing that defined me or to influence the way in which we related to each other; because I didn't want her to treat me any differently than she would anyone else, or feel she had to tiptoe around me; because I didn't want to leave myself any leeway to use my condition as an excuse or fallback for any abnormal but unrelated behaviour. As time passed, I fell into a kind of complacency, taking the incident-and-episode-free first few months of our relationship as proof enough that there was no need to bother.

One of the benefits of our long-distance relationship has been that shielding the most colourful manifestations of the condition from Aiyla has been easy, but at the same time it means that I've denied her a fair impression of what it might be like to live with a Bipolar partner. Now, based on the evidence of symptoms that I've accumulated these past few days – speaking to myself, distractedness, the overload of manic energy in dire need of offloading – I have a feeling that might be about to change.

I call her after my session on the wall. She's on her bed, watching a show on her laptop while petting one of the four stray kittens she's taken in over the past week.

'I think,' I tell her, after edging the conversation away from recent developments in the Kadiköy cat population on to why I've been climbing so much these past few days, subtly preparing the ground for what will follow, 'I'm manic.'

'Okayyyyy,' she says, shifting the mewling kitten from her chest onto the bed as a statement of intent. 'What have you noticed so far?'

'My heart rate's up. My hands are shaky. I feel like I could run twenty marathons and still be as fresh as a daisy. Green looks greater than it should do. Light blue, too. I'm too distracted to work and when I force myself to sit down, words look like hieroglyphics. And I've been panicking about this whole reopening business,' I say, opting to leave out the bit about talking to myself, for now. 'I might just be overreacting, but . . .'

Am I overreacting? There's always doubt, always second-guessing the origin of certain behaviours, and questions about whether I can ever do anything entirely uninfluenced by the condition.

'Have you been having heart palpitations?'

'A bit, yeah.'

'Anxiety.'

'Yep.'

'What about shopping?'

'Shopping?'

'That's one of the few non-subjective flags, right?'

'Well, yeah, but . . .'

'Have you done any?'

'Nah, none.'

'Sure?'

'Yeah, sure.'

'Open your email.'

I flip open my laptop and open my email. There, in my inbox, I find four pieces of irrefutable evidence, unopened, at the top of the page.

I click on the emails.

'Cigars,' I say. 'Twenty of them. And squeaky toys. And a camming device for climbing. And a trash-grabber for Giuseppina.'

'Squeaky toys?'

'For Vincenzo, my sister's dachshund, and Rufus.'

'Okay, what about the cigars? You don't even smoke any more.'

'I know, but I thought Matteo and Lucia and Michele and Gaia and I could smoke them at the top of all the climbs we're going to do when we're able to go climbing with friends again at the end of May.'

'Okay, you said you were panicking. What's making you panic?'

'The end of the lockdown. I'm scared. I don't know when I'll see you or Ma or Pa or Cath again, and the world we're going to be seeing each other in's going to be shit.'

'Is the world shit now?'

'Yeah, of course.'

'What makes you feel that's true?'

'The deaths. The unemployment. The millions of people who're gonna go hungry. Trump. Bolsonaro. Republicans. Tories. The *Centrodestra*. Conspiracy theorists. It's like all the ingredients that make a life worth living have been taken out of the pot and we've been left with shit croutons.'

'Okay. I understand the deaths, the hunger and the unemployment. But tell me more about the ingredients that make life worth living.'

'Freedom. Connection with others. Adventure. Love. And then a little more freedom. I mean, I'm not about to round up my friends and go storm the mayor's office or anything, but the world has become smaller, no doubt about it. The possibilities that were there have shrunk. Variety isn't the spice of life; possibility is.'

'How does that make you feel?'

'Shite.'

'Can you be more specific?'

'Really shite. Like there's no future. Like I'm in a room and there's no door.'

'And do you feel like you're rejecting your feelings or welcoming them?'

'I feel like I don't have a choice. They're there. They're real.'

'Okay. What would make it feel less shite? Right now. If you could do anything you wanted . . .'

'I don't know.'

'Nothing?'

'Not unless someone's offering to take out Trump and Boris and start taxing every multibillionaire on the planet their fair share so we can feed and look after—'

'Something more realistic, maybe.'

'Okay. A climb. A big, long, satisfying climb. Dirty hands. Shredded fingers. Peeing in the woods. Sunburned arms. Wedging a cam* into a perfect crack. The clipping sound of a carabiner. Running the rope over the top of my forefinger and into a quickdraw† after a sketchy move. Sitting on the top of a route at the end of the day feeling like I've conquered the world, and then coming down and having pizza with the gang and sharing the stories of our climbs and everything being perfect because all of us know we're exactly where we should be.'

I've closed my eyes to wallow in the imagery conjured by

---

* A spring-loaded device that can be jammed into rock fissures and then attached to a rope with a sling and carabiner for safety.
† A pair of carabiners connected by semi-rigid material: one is clipped into a bolted hanger (or cam or nut) and the rope passed through the other to reduce the distance of any fall.

my words as I speak them. I expect Aiyla to be yawning the-
atrically or tapping her fingers on her cheek when I open them
again, feigning disapproval but betraying her amusement with
a wry but tolerant, long-suffering smile. If I've really overdone
it she'll throw in a facepalm for good measure or be making
the T-for-timeout gesture with her hands.

There's no facepalm, no smile. Her dark eyes gaze out
humourlessly from the screen.

'What?' I say.

'I was kinda hoping I'd figure in there somewhere.'

Shite.

'You do, obviously. Only I know it's going to be a long time
before we see each other again. Going climbing feels like a
more realistic possibility than hopping on a plane to Turkey.
In the near future, anyway.'

'Right.'

'And if you were living here, then it wouldn't be an issue.
I mean, we'd be seeing each other all the—'

'What? In Sondrio?'

'Well, yeah. I mean, we haven't talked about it as an option
yet, have we?'

'Do we have to?'

'Well, I thought that, maybe—'

'Kieran . . .'

'What?'

'How could I possibly continue my career in a place where
I don't speak the language and there are no universities within
a two-hour radius?'

'I just thought, you know, it was like you said about your
clients – that all this might have made you rethink things and

not want to spend twelve hours a day stuck in an office and commuting. I know it wouldn't be easy, but think about it – we could get a little house in the mountains and I'd do my usual stuff or get a job as a forester or mountain guide, and you could do your sessions online. I could teach you to ski and climb and we could eat pizza every night. And cannoli. And bresaola. We'd grow stuff in the garden like Fausto. We could get goats and a dog and—'

'Cats?'

A whisper of a smile rises at the corners of her mouth.

'Well, that's a bit of a highball counter, but I'd be willing to consider it if you'd be willing to submit to the rest of the outlined conditions.'

'Let me think about it.'

Lockdown Day 56

I'm not there yet, but it's coming. I can't tell if it's going to be a full-blown episode or just a quickie. My forecasting on internal weather has been off since this thing began and unable to keep up with the erratic fluctuations of the past few weeks in particular. Normally I pick up on things in meditation, or when I'm in the mountains, or I can take a more statistical approach by weighing the duration and intensity of the initial, shorter cycles to predict subsequent cycles, but this time there's no pattern.

It feels lonely. Very lonely. Though talking to Aiyla or any other psychiatric specialist can help, the impossibility of conveying the experience accurately and the absence of common ground makes it feel like your ground's an island.

I didn't meet anyone else with Bipolar 1 until three or four years ago. His name is Andy, a young guy from my village in Scotland who works with his dad in construction a few months every year then takes off to travel in South America and Asia. Ma'd met his mum in a café somewhere and they got talking, as Ma is wont, and arranged for us to meet, like a playdate for kids who share not the same hobby or school but the same succubus at the controls of their neurochemical command centres. I'd been sceptical, but it turned out to be one of the most encouraging experiences I've ever had, and the start of a valuable and meaningful friendship. We first met when I was giving a talk at the local library about mountaineering and life in Italy. Around fifty people showed up, but I somehow picked him out in the crowd within a minute of arriving. At the end of the talk, we introduced ourselves and went outside for a 'quick smoke break' that lasted three hours. It was the first time I'd felt that someone had understood me when I'd spoken about episodes and the day-to-day struggles of being Bipolar, as if we shared not only a set of symptoms but also a language. Now, every time I return home, we camp out under the gazebo in his garden for all-day decompression sessions and take long walks along the beach, recounting how we've fared in our latest stint in the world of Normals and sharing our experiences with meds, therapists and the fluctuations in our mental firmware. The most transformational thing to come out of it has been learning that many of the things I once thought unique to the way I experienced Bipolar were ones he shared, and most of the fears I harboured regarding my moods and prospects for negotiating life could be disarmed by simply giving voice to them, airing them out instead of leaving them to lignify in my head.

Here in Sondrio I have one less fellow sufferer to turn to.

I also have no doctor, no Ma, no Pa, no Cath, no Aiyla, no anybody else who could lend an understanding ear and confirm or disavow my suspicion that my behaviour these past days has contained more than a marginal whiff of a manic episode in the making.

I can't stop crying today. This morning, it was thinking about Giuseppina's daughter in Novara, Beatrice, who normally visits every weekend but hasn't been able to make it back in two months and is stuck in her apartment with a broken metatarsal in her foot from a dishwasher accident and without her partner, who got trapped in Veneto before lockdown. Then it was thinking of the kids I used to teach, about the effect all this is bound to have on them and countless others for years to come. Then thinking of tomorrow and the uncertainty about what things will be like on the other side of lockdown, no matter how watered down it seems our version of reopening will be.

The crying thing's new. It comes mostly without warning or due cause. I'll be going about my normal business – at my computer, making coffee, showering, doing housework – and find the tears welling in my eyes, usually as a result of something that at any other time wouldn't warrant a reaction. I can only guess the cumulative trauma and unease of the past few months has shifted my emotional baseline.

I'm feeling itchy inside by 4 p.m. and go climbing early, even though the sun is ferocious and the holds almost too hot to touch. I put in my twenty-five traverses on the Dusk Wall and then another fifteen or so on the Scorpion Wall and Indecent Exposure, upping the stakes by allowing myself to use only two fingers from each hand, then one finger, then one hand only. When I'm done with those, I'm still buzzing, so fumble around on the now ivy-infested Dirty Wall for twenty minutes before returning to the Dusk Wall, determined to tire myself out before bed.

I'm still climbing at 8 p.m. and decide to call Aiyla.

The call starts off normally enough: pleasantries, I-miss-yous, questions about each other's days and suchlike. Then I break loose, off-script, diverging from the sanctioned, tactful line of conversation I'd promised myself I'd stick to when I'd decided to call.

I've been ranting at her for over half an hour, working myself into a lather, before I get onto one of my manic self's favourite topics: *On Why We Should All Be Screaming in the Streets*, a lengthy litany on the awesomeness and absurdity of human consciousness.

'Are you okay, baby?' Aiyla asks, interrupting me.

By now I'm pacing the lower tier of the garden beneath the magnolia, having shifted round to the other side of the house to get a better view of the gossamer tendrils of cloud in the moonlight above the tops of Pizzo di Rodes and Pizzo Meriggio.

'What? Yeah. Let's go up on the mountain and look at it. The stars and stuff. The air. The leaves. I'll put my shoes on. Then we can see how magical it all is and understand how fucking ridiculous it is that there's anything there at all. Why don't we see that? Why ... wait ...'

I do a forward roll on the grass. When I stand there's a small, irate face screaming at me on my phone.

'Kieran! *Kieran!*'

'Yeah.'

'I need you to do something for me.'

'Yeah, sure. What?'

'Go back inside.'

'But—'

'Baby, please just go back inside.'

'But you didn't see the—'

'*Please*, just do it.'

'Okay. We can come back later.'

I go back inside. My chest is puffed and my body feels electrically charged. I have the feeling of having done something I should be very proud of but can't be sure what.

'Just sit down,' Aiyla says.

'Nah. I'm not tired. I should go climbing! They say we can't see our friends for two weeks and even if we can the crags will be dirty with all the Covid hands that have been all over them. *I can't wait two weeks.* I can take my self-belay device and rope and go to the crag at Sirta or Sassella. Actually, fuck it, I don't even need the rope. I've done all of those climbs thousands of times and never fallen once.'

'Kieran, *please*!'

'Okay, okay.'

Eventually I sit and continue my rant from the couch. Some part of me is aware that she's not taking this well and I manage to calm myself enough to convince her that I'm not as gone as she thinks, channelling my Normal Me as much as possible and resisting every urge to moonwalk, forward roll, rush back outside and howl at the moon, tell her all about the ontology of mountains and how I'm fairly sure quantum physics will soon dispel any remaining notion that we might have so much as a grain of free will.

We talk for hours. Around midnight, I pretend to be tired and end the call, telling her I'm going to sleep, which I should probably do, but don't. Instead, I shift my chair to the living room window and sit in my boxer shorts gazing out into the liquid night, spellbound by everything in general but nothing in particular, smitten by each and every one of the stimuli arising and receding in any given second. The world outside's a mess; that which surrounds me is a harlequin chandelier glittering with every colour, cuteness and quaintness imaginable; every second is the bringer of a brand-new cavalcade of sensory curios upon which my eyes, ears, nose, skin and every other bit of me feeds in a euphoric lovesick frenzy until long after the first blush of sunrise announces itself upon the flanks of the Orobie.

A warning flag's waving somewhere in the rear-view mirror of my mind's eye, exhorting stitches in time – *been here before*'s and suchlike – but already its counsel dims in the distance. This is the compensation, you see. Damages for injuries sustained – the non-deductible counterweight to the net and sundry cost of living. While I'd never wish the rest of it on anyone, this – *this* – is something for which I'd fight to the death should any cure-toting doctor appear and try to take it away from me.

Lockdown Day 57

Monday, 4 May. What am I going to do today?

There are no fireworks. No parties. No celebrations. No tooting of horns and blaring music.

The city looks bashful in the morning sun, as though

regretting all the clamorous calls for reopening now that the time has come.

One of the greatest problems I've experienced since moving here has been a kid-in-a-candy-store kind of indecision when it comes to deciding what to do every weekend. Early in the week, I draw up ten-item lists of potential climbs or mountaineering routes, taking into account avalanche forecasts, sun exposure, altitude gain and difficulty, and spend most of my week debating the options. Today, though doubts still remain as to what we can and can't do, that indecision is back.

What *is* clear – or less nebulous, to be more precise – is that whatever I do, I have to do it alone.

I draw up a shortlist of options:

1. Climb Corna Mara. It's a 8,210-foot hike from my apartment to the summit, around a twelve-hour return trip.
2. Wander in the vineyards above town until tired.
3. Take a stroll through town to see what humans other than Giuseppina and her family look like and get the lie of the land.

Option one is appealing, but I'm unsure if my knee's up to it – the 12-hour trip could easily become a 24-hour one if the knee bails on me anywhere near the top. Option two feels a little tame. Option three feels overwhelming but curiously appealing.

I decide on a combo of options two and three – an easy break-in to start the acclimatisation.

First, I have to stop crying. I've been at it all morning.

Today's triggers are a friend from the US who's been trapped in India since mid-March, news that the mother of a neighbour who died of the virus also died of it two days ago, and the ringing of the church bells, which sound like mothers feeding their children.

Bipolar often feels like a misnomer. Agony and ecstasy are not mutually exclusive. The poles meet and merge, cycles turn within cycles. Ups coalesce with downs. Moods are a cross-pollination of every feeling on the spectrum of human emotion. Often, the joy is more agonising than the despair, and the despair spangled with exquisitely raw, visceral beauty.

I've called Aiyla to apologise for last night. It was a pro forma apology, one scripted by the me who's done such wrongs a million times before, and not the one who still, at this moment, despite all the tears and hypersensitivity, feels altogether peachy.

Yesterday, my self-awareness – my 'meta' – was about as low as it can be. There's a scale, and in the course of any episode my meta can run the full gamut, from entirely unwitting to a fully cognisant, third-person view of whatever my first person might be up to. Today I'm better. High but also mindful and aware of my lack of awareness, which is about as good as it gets. A solid 9 on the meta-ometer. This being so, I know that, before I do anything else, to make the rest of the day safe – from a Bipolar if not a Covid point of view – I need to go running.

I go to the vineyards above town.

I'd expected a Black Friday-style mob to have descended on every square inch of unenclosed space but pass nobody between Giuseppina's gate and the second tier of the vineyards, some twenty minutes later.

I see him approaching in the distance: a man, walking with a slight limp and stoop, his hands clasped behind his back. He looks up when I come within 50 metres of him and I somehow understand that I'm the first person he's seen since reopening, too.

'*Ciao!*' he says, his voice gurgling enthusiastically.

'*Ciao!*' I reply.

'*Ciao, ciao!*' he repeats.

Before I'm ten steps past him, my legs go weak and tears are rolling off my cheeks onto my bare chest. I force myself to carry on.

The valley is aching with life. Everything appears more vibrant, in high contrast, rich. My eyes are drawn repeatedly to the side of the path, where occasional shocks of herb robert, rock soapwort and alpine rose have sprung between the cobbled stones of the path and the retaining walls of the vineyard. I loop up onto the second tier. There, I see a couple with a pram approaching in the distance and decide to turn around, just to be safe. I see the man from before again on the way down. He's turned around, too, and as I pass and greet him a second time I get the same weakness, the same surge of emotion, and have to stop. I double over, pretending to be out of breath, while tears and laughter flood out of me simultaneously.

After my jog, I go down to the pharmacy to stock up on masks. While I'm browsing the limited options, I hear a close approximation of my name from the other side of the counter.

'I'm surprised you haven't started climbing again yet,' says the bespectacled, masked, white-coated figure stood at the counter beside a sign illustrating appropriate mask usage.

It's Giancarlo, the head pharmacist, an outstanding climber who put up dozens of first ascents on new sport routes* throughout the valley in the 1990s and bolted the crag at Fusine with a friend so they'd have somewhere to climb in the shade in the summer.

'I didn't think it was possible yet,' I say.

'Of course it is!'

For the first time I have mask envy. He's wearing one of the fancy moulded affairs with the little filter button in the middle. No sooner has this passed than a second, more potent blow is struck as I glance down at the counter and clock traces of climbing chalk around the edges of his nails. *The bastard.*

'All you have to do,' he says, 'is fill out your *autocertificazione*, then you can go anywhere. Sure, someone might kick up a stink if you're too close to your partner, but if you arrive in separate cars there shouldn't be any problem. Just don't tell anyone I said so if you get caught. If you want, I'll be at Fusine with David and a few others this afternoon after four.'

I tell him I might come, but by the time I've left the store I already know I won't go. The logistics entailed in keeping things clean and safe while using the same rope, the same quickdraws, the same belay device and, of course, the same

---

* 'Sport' climbing refers to climbing on single-pitch routes, which are usually 10–35 metres long and have fixed hangers in the rock through which quick-draws can be clipped for safety. While a bit of an all-rounder, I consider myself a 'trad' (traditional) and alpine climber, above all else, but sport climbing is, for almost all climbers, the most practical way of training for everything else. Each of the four main types of climbing – bouldering, sport, trad and alpine – requires very different skill sets and appeals to a different mentality. In the words of Luigi: 'Boulderers are problem-solving technicians, sport climbers are gymnasts, trad climbers are engineers, alpine climbers are adventurers. All of us are madmen and poets.'

rock, make my mind spin. Supposing just one of the proposed five who'll be there has the virus, by the time we're finished there's a good chance all of us will.

Thus far, Day 57 has felt very much like Day 56, only with a little more legroom. The British Airways of quarantine as opposed to the Ryanair.

In town, the division of those who have gardens or balconies from those who don't is highly visible, revealed by a straight 50:50 split between pasty-white and tanned. Everyone's masked, everyone's doing their distancing, everyone looks slightly dazed and edgy. Nothing's open yet, but people appear to have somewhere to go.

In the afternoon, I burn a batch of scones while distracted by another attempt at work, then set off for a longer walk up the hill behind town.

I call Aiyla as soon as I'm off the road and into the vineyards.

'Yesterday was scary,' she says.

I know yesterday was scary. I'm still too high to empathise fully, but aware that the gap between the me she's known for the past two years and the one she saw last night is a big one.

'I've never seen you like that before.'

'I know,' I say, trying as much as possible to channel whatever non-manic part of me remains behind the part that wants to ask her to dance to David Bowie's 'Magic Dance' like in the good old days, before our reality took a turn for the tits-up and tragic, 'but circumstances are kinda extenuating, Aiyla.'

'I just don't get it. It was the day before the end of quarantine. Just three hours away from freedom.'

'Bipolar isn't the best timekeeper,' I say, 'and doesn't really keep abreast or give a hoot about the news. And just because some official in Rome says we can leave our homes, it doesn't mean the virus has suddenly gone or there aren't a quarter of a million people dead and we haven't just spent the past two months of our lives cooped up in our homes going batshit-crazy.'

'I know, but . . .'

There's a but?

'There's a "but"?'

'I just worry, you know. I'm a psychologist, so of course I understand that this has been a shitty time for you, but I get to freak out too, you know.'

'Of course. I'd be worried if you *weren't* worried.'

'No,' she says, 'I mean I'm worried about *us*. Our future. It's not the way you are when you're high, but what you say. All you do is gush about climbing and mountains and Sondrio. It's impossible for me to see where I'll fit into your life.'

'Those are my passions, Aiyla. You know that. They're more than that, even. They're the things that keep me alive and sane and make this whole aliveness and sanity business worthwhile. It's natural that I should start waxing lyrical about them just at the time when my sanity's under threat, don't you think? And I place you in the same category, by the way. I only prattle on about them so freely to you because I've never seen it as a zero-sum game – there's never been any question in my head about there being plenty of room for both of you, and I never thought it had to be one or the other.'

'I get that, but what if we have a family somewhere down the line?'

'Eh? Climbers have kids. Look at Tommy Caldwell!'

'Kieran, you're hardly Tommy Caldwell.'

'A low blow, but an accurate one, granted.'

I'm on the path on the bottom-most tier of the vineyards, where the rows of plants end abruptly above the village of Colda, a one-street affair of slate-built houses attached to Sondrio's north-eastern periphery. A pair of scruffy pinschers at the back of one of the gardens are yapping their balls off at me as I pass. Every chaffinch, swallow and swift in Italy seems to have convened in the trees flanking the path to protest the reappearance of humans. I've no sooner passed out of earshot of my animal assailants than a troupe of chatty joggers arrives behind me, forcing me to cut up one of the rows of vines to find a quieter spot on the second tier.

'I'm just trying to think logically,' Aiyla continues. 'I'm not saying any of this because I don't understand how passionate you people are; it's because I *do* understand. When you say all these things and start saying how bored you are with work and how, if you could, you'd just spend your life climbing all the time, it's natural that a few flags should start waving, right? I mean, what if, somewhere down the line, you just say "Fuck it" and decide to follow your dreams and ambitions instead of . . .'

'. . . holing myself up in an office and waiting patiently for death but consoling myself with the thought that I bought my kids the new iPhone they wanted? Spiriting away my condition so I can get down to some good old, trouble-free, old-fashioned homemaking?'

'You know that's not what I meant.'

'Then what *do* you mean?'

'Are we gonna be able to make this work? I'm not like Lucia or Giulia or Gaia or any of your other friends. I'm not a climber.'

'You're precisely the same girl I fell in love with when we met, and that's how I like you. Why would I feel any differently now? And it's the same with me – I was a penniless, Bipolar writer with a climbing habit when you met me, and I'm still a penniless, Bipolar writer with a climbing habit now. What's changed? Yeah, sometimes I get pissy about my job, but who doesn't? And I don't do it because it's ideal – far from it; just because it's the only one I've found so far that makes it possible for me to manage things. Look, if you want a neurotypical guy, one who'll be an emotionally stable, strait-laced, archetypal provider for our future family, then God, there are safer bets to be found. If that's who will make you happy, then I'll give you my blessing to go find one.'

'That's not what I want.'

'Then help me understand.'

'Can I ask you something – something kinda big?'

I've taken a seat on the dry-stone wall above the second tier. A dog walker I didn't see approaching has stopped to ogle me from the path below while waiting for his aged papillon, some 20 metres behind and taking a shit dead-centre of the path, to catch up with him. His mask makes it impossible to tell if he's smiling or not. I wave; he doesn't wave back. I nudge myself back into the enclosure of the vines and wait until the man's shuffled out of earshot before replying.

'Go ahead.'

'Why have you never had kids? Is it something you've ever thought about?'

'Yeah, of course. It's always been one of my biggest dreams.'

'Why didn't it happen with any of your exes?'

'I wasn't ready. Not in the way that other people say they

aren't ready but because I *really* wasn't ready. Until recently, I'd spent my whole life fighting to eke out a space in which I could get by in the world, just trying to cover the things at the base of that pyramid thingy you told me about. Kids were always higher up the pyramid. I couldn't hold down a job. I couldn't even hold down friends. I couldn't really think about anything besides making it from one day to the next. *That* was success for me. And it still is, kinda. Before this virus shit hit, though, I'd got past it. I had a semi–reliable job that I didn't hate so much that I'm likely to quit or get myself fired from soon. I had friends. I was healthy. I had the base of the pyramid covered. And hopefully I'll get back there again soon, assuming there aren't too many more Covids in the pipeline.'

'So, you'd consider it?'

The sky's pinkening to the west. The mournful peal of the church bells in the village of Montagna seems to percolate in the gummy, humid night air. I try to think of something else to talk about, but nothing comes to me.

'Kieran?'

'Well . . . yeah.'

'That wasn't convincing.'

'Eh? What are you getting at?'

'Look, I know when you're holding something back. You're doing it now. You can tell me. If you want to, that is. And if you don't, that's okay too.'

She's right. In the minute I spend mentally editing and redacting a series of potential answers that might get her off my case, I realise something. Beneath the stock replies I've always given to Ma, aunties, and anyone else who's bothered asking there's a grimmer truth that—

Before I know if I can come out with it, I've come out with it:

'It's hereditary, Aiyla. There's every chance they'd be like me.'

The searching look that animated her eyes just a few minutes ago is gone in an instant, replaced by a startling tenderness. She doesn't move for a few seconds, and I think the screen has frozen, but then I hear the ululating voice of the muezzin calling the evening *salat* outside her window.

'Kieran,' she finally says, 'that's horrible. You—'

'I need to finish. This isn't easy to say. I know how much you want kids. But I have to be honest. Last night was tame. I'd been stable for a long time before this happened, yes, but what you saw last night was nothing compared to how bad it can be. And I have no clue whether or not it'll be that bad again. I know it's horrible, but the reason I've never even come close to having kids is because I wouldn't want anyone to have to go through the same shit I have. I'm better now than I've ever been, but I haven't had enough time to enjoy being me without the shit to know if it would be an act of kindness or cruelty to set someone else up for the same thing. I'm still discovering whether it's worthwhile. For now, it is, but I feel like I'm in a bubble here. In Sondrio, I mean. It took me fucking ages to find this place and if Brexit buggers things up, or Ma or Pa get sick, or we decide to live somewhere else, I'm scared things will go back to the way they were before. And what if my kids aren't lucky enough to find their own Sondrio? I'd feel responsible for everything they experience, wherever else they happen to be. I know you want to have kids and I'd hate myself for standing in your way. I wish I could just vanish my

265

condition and say yeah, I'm in, but I can't. Not yet. I might get there, eventually, but it will take time.'

Lockdown Day 58

Day two of freedom.

I get a text from Lucia in the morning warning me not to go climbing. A few of her climber friends were fined yesterday at the crag in Ponte, where I went with her and Matteo two days before lockdown. Sporting activity, the police told her friends, is allowed only as long as it's done alone or with family members.

I've stopped crying today – evidence that all that fresh air yesterday did me good.

Before breakfast, I hear a vehicle parking up on the lane outside the house, behind the Dusk Wall, and then voices outside the kitchen window. The vehicle is a little truck with a huge liquid-container attached to the back, the voices those of hazmat-suited vineyard workers brandishing hoses attached to the container, working their way through the rows of vines, spraying them with insecticide. I lean out the window to see if any of them fancy a chat, but realise I'm only trying to distract myself from thoughts about my argument last night with Aiyla and the subsequent texts that did little to remedy the blows we'd dealt each other during our phone call.

I replay the conversation and our texts in my head throughout the morning while migrating back and forth between the kitchen window, my desk and my climbing cupboard in a soupy, stunned stupor. I can understand her. I've always felt like I should come with a warning of the 'this product contains (is?) nuts' variety found on food packaging. I maybe should have done more to prepare her for the inevitable shock of when she first witnessed an episode, no matter how tame the other night was in the scale of things. But I'd been scared of scaring her off, too, chastened by too many relationships halted in their tracks by the mere admission of the 'baggage' I was bringing into them and, of course, hadn't predicted that my condition's hiatus in hostilities would be curtailed by a pandemic and sixty-day quarantine that would create the optimal conditions to trigger symptoms. Maybe part of me was also guilty of wishful thinking, hoping that my newfound happiness would be so thorough as to overrule my mental miswiring and I'd never have to tell her how bad it could be because the bad would never come.

The thought of losing her terrifies me, but it's a relief that it's out. It's part of me, this; part of the deal. Not the best deal, maybe, but the best deal I have to offer.

We speak again later in the morning. Stiltedly. Dodging around the details of last night's quarrel. It feels like something might be broken but it's too soon to tell.

I manage to get in five hours of work by lunchtime – the first time I've managed this in over a week. When I'm done, I scoot out to the big supermarket outside town, not because I'm short on supplies just yet, but so I can get a look at the crag at Sassella and see if anyone's climbing yet. If it were allowed, or if any of the valley's climbers really thought the more favourable reading of the *decreto* was legit, Sassella would be packed.

The crag's empty.

Cazzo.

After showering and shelving my groceries, I get dressed,

fill a backpack with 10 kilos of weights, and head to the vines above town, hoping to put in 600 metres of ascent so I can better gauge my cardio fitness and whether my knee's in good enough shape to take me up a mountain in the coming days. Joining Luigi and Co. for a crag-climbing session might be a risk too far, but a solo climb in the mountains might soon be one I'm willing to take, knowing that the likely reward will be getting myself out of this thing safely.

I walk for two hours without stopping, ending in the forest below Corna Mara. My altimeter tells me I've done 987 metres of ascent, much more than I'd planned, and my knee has only given the odd twinge of discomfort. With every step I've taken upwards, I've allowed myself to start believing that the nightmare's nearing its end. Soon, it seems, control over my own well-being will be back in my own hands.

On the way down, I veer west and rejoin the top path in the vineyard above the village of Ponchiera. Half a kilometre or so before the village, I see a small red tractor parked above a U-shaped gulley, at the centre of which is a vegetable plot. I see the tractor's owner working among the plot of greens, turning the soil between the rows with a backhoe.

I met the man, Eugenio, a few years ago when passing the same spot and again the day before my last visit to Istanbul, when I went walking up there to do the same thing I was doing now – test my knee and gauge how soon I'd need an operation. We ended up sitting above his plot for a full afternoon, then returned to his house in Montagna for dinner with his daughter and wife, who'd sent me home with a five-kilo round of *bitto* cheese, a bottle of homemade grappa and two bottles of wine from the vineyard, casually countering my confessions of being allergic to cheese and teetotal with a chuckle, stomp of her foot and a hearty slap on my shoulder.

He's the first person I've seen not wearing a mask and is dressed in the same soiled corduroy trousers, off-white vest and bedraggled, buttonless plaid shirt as the last time I saw him.

'The wanderer returns!' he says when he looks up from his work and sees me shuffling down the steep dirt track above the plot. 'How was Iran?'

'Turkey?'

'Same thing, no?'

'It seems like a lifetime ago.'

'Yes, I imagine it does.'

'How have you been?'

He pulls on his belt and spits into the soil at his feet.

'Same as ever. I hear the rest of you have had a bit of a holiday.'

'Something like that, yeah.'

'*Beati voi!* I have 16 hectares of vineyard to look after, then this *orto* and the orchards. I haven't had a day off in sixty-four years! Nobody told the grapes or the spinach or the apples or the salad there was any virus going around. Came just the same as ever. It's like having a million children – all of them needing to be fed and watered all the time. Why are you laughing?'

'Want a hand?'

'And I thought you were just going to stand there yapping all day. Grab that hoe next to the wall.'

I make a start on the row below the one Eugenio's working on. We work in silence, except for when he's saying *'Puttana!'* to the rocks that get in the way of his hoe as he swings it into the soil, or he thinks I've dug too deep or got too close to the plants and lets me know with a gruff call over his shoulder. I lose myself in thought until, maybe twenty minutes later, we meet at the end of our respective rows. Eugenio stops, angles the hoe into his armpit and props himself against it, taking a handkerchief from his shirt pocket to mop down his brow and pat beneath his ruddied jowls.

'What's wrong with you today, anyway? Your head's in the air. Girl troubles?'

'Good guess.'

'The Turkish lass?'

'Yep.'

'*Ma va!* You showed me a picture of her last time. A girl like that doesn't cause any problems that aren't worth tolerating.'

'She's great, yeah, but it's starting to look like we might want different things.'

'We have a saying here: *Moglie e buoi di paesi tuoi* [Wives and cows from your own land], but I've never much believed in it. Any man who doesn't believe all the world is his land is a poor one. That's your problem there.'

'I don't follow.'

'You're a mountain man, aren't you?'

'I suppose I am, yeah.'

'And her?'

'Not a mountain woman.'

'Well, there you go. My daughter's one of them now, too. Married a Milanese. Comes home once a month for the weekend. Think I understand her? No. But it works both ways. I could have retired twelve years ago, but instead I'm here, breaking my back over kilometre after kilometre of fruit and vegetables that'll give me no thanks for it. And you, you're here too, standing in my dirt and manure, making a mess of my *orto* when you could be back home eating dinner and playing games on your computer or watching shit on the telly. And tomorrow I imagine you'll be somewhere molesting a big rock, shredding your skin and shitting yourself, or up in the mountains, arse-deep in snow, skiting about on ice, freezing your nuts off and calling it *divertimento*. Think they understand that? No chance.'

He spits into the earth again and re-wipes his brow.

'Get what I'm saying?' he asks.

'Not really.'

'Mountains are magical places, *ragazzo*, but they aren't everything. Know how many lads like you I've known over the years? *Un sacco* [a bagful]. *È una tragedia.*'

'*Morti?*'

'Not dead, single. And lonely. They're as old as me and never had any more meaningful a relationship than with the *tizio* [guy] whose *culo* [arse] they're staring at going up their climbs ahead of them. I see them now, teaching or climbing with young lasses half their age, angling for you know what. Embarrassing.'

He punctuates the thought by spitting into the soil and swinging the blade of the hoe into a patch of soil he's already furrowed.

'Hate to be the one to break it to you, *caro*,' he continues, 'but *hai vinto la lotteria* – you're punching above your weight. You're not getting any younger, you've a nose on you nearly as big as mine, and you've been in those same grungy trousers and shirt every time I've seen you. I know nothing of the girl's character, but don't let your passion for one thing rule out the rest of them. Maybe it's time you did some thinking about whether or not you're *esagerando* [being over the top] – you wouldn't be the first of your lot, I assure you. Look at my plants. *Cazzo*, I'd rather be another 1,000 metres up this mountain, but I know not one of these plants would make it through a winter. Then what? What I'm saying is, you have to decide how far you're willing to come down to let things grow; the girl has to decide how far up she's willing to go to breathe the fresh air and live. If the distance between you is too big, then you'd be best moving on, but I haven't met a soul yet who wouldn't have benefited from making *paesi suoi* a tad bigger rather than a tad smaller.'

I call Ma when I get home. She's been out of bed for a few days now and is in the kitchen when she answers.

'I was out for a walk this morning,' she says, proud of herself. 'I got along to the library then had to turn back, but I did well, I think. They still won't let me go in for one of these tests so I'm wearing a mask, just to keep the neighbours happy. It was soaking wet when I got home, though, so I must have had it on the wrong way around. What a dafty, eh? Did I tell you our new kettle and toaster came this morning? They're lovely! Kind of a baby-blue like your car. I was telling Moira over the wall – do you know they don't even wash their shopping after they've been to the supermarket? I was telling her that ... Oh, I forgot to ask you – how's it been with the reopening?'

The 'reopening' has been anticlimactic and done little to inspire hope that 2 June, when the last part of reopening takes place, will be much better.

Beyond the daily walks, my climbing buddies blithely

disregarding social-distancing and mask-wearing protocols on their resumption of attendance at our local crags (*'il Covid se ne è già andato'* – 'Covid's already gone'), and a little more foot traffic in the streets below my apartment, 'normality' doesn't feel much like normality. I still feel as though I have one foot in quarantine, one in the lee of the new status quo we're tiptoeing into.

In many ways, it's worse. While locked up in our homes, we didn't see the oddity. Outside existed as a world-in-the-offing – a Schrödinger's world, of sorts; now, the memory of the cat that went into the box jars with the cold, unfamiliar reality of the one now before us.

If not 2 June, or whenever restrictions are fully lifted, then when, I ask myself, will this feel over for me? What would constitute an end? When they find a vaccine? A cure? When I finally get to see Aiyla, or my family, or my friends again? None of them are likely to happen any time soon.

Bugger it. Tomorrow, I'm going climbing.

Lockdown Day 59

Preparation for climbing is almost as much a part of the joy as the act itself. If you don't have a passion for the process – the endless maintenance and checking and preparation of ropes and other gear – then it's hard to become enamoured with the rest of it.

I remember the reverence with which Pa went about his gear prep when I was a kid, explicitly because there was something so kookily intense and obsessive about it that it merited isolation in the archives of memory. There's a large walk-in airing cupboard at the top of the stairs at home, stuffed to the brim with enough rucksacks, tents, sleeping bags, helmets, ice axes, crampons, ropes, camming devices, nuts, slings, quick-draws and belay devices for a team of at least six climbers. The day before climbing trips, Pa would hole himself up in there to pick out everything he'd need for the proposed route, deaf to whatever was going on elsewhere in the house, and usually for far longer than seemed necessary or reasonable. He'd lay it all out carefully on the landing and go through each piece of gear individually, inspecting and admiring, before finally packing it away in his rucksack. I'd catch him in the cupboard at other times, too: when he returned from a stressful day at work and hadn't been able to go to the climbing wall in Edinburgh or the local crags at Dairsie and Aberdour; on breaks from his laptop after he started working from home; whenever he had an argument with Ma; or whenever our football team was playing our local rivals and the tension got too much.

I don't sleep a wink. I try to stay in bed to make sure I'm in good enough shape to get in the kind of long, satisfying, soul-and-sanity-restoring session I've been dreaming about, but by 3 a.m. my brain's already on the wall and wondering why my body's not there with it.

I go into my gear cupboard straight from bed, feeling like a child sneaking into the pantry after the adults have gone to sleep. I take my 80-metre rope from the padded hanger and 'flake' it out on the floor to eliminate kinks and coils that may later prevent it running smoothly. After flaking, I recoil the rope in neat loops to make it easy to carry from the park-ing area to the crag, and lay it by the front door. Next, I go through my gear sling and pick out all the hardware I'll need for the climbs I plan on doing. Today I'll be climbing at a sport-climbing crag where the routes have bolted hangers that allow me to protect the climb every few metres by clipping in my rope with quickdraws, so I need to take twelve quick-draws, a belay device for abseils, four carabiners, two slings, my harness, and the self-belay device that lets me 'rope-solo', i.e. climb without a partner but with a mechanical aid that will arrest a fall. I try to be methodical but start dropping things in my excitement.

While one of my regular climbing groups is refusing to climb until it's safe and legal to do so, and the other is confined to crags hidden from the roadside and the prying eyes of vil-lagers who might object and inform the authorities, using the self-belay device means I should be able to resume climbing, safely and legally, at any crag I choose.

I choose to climb at Sirta, an 80-metre-high, 200-metre-wide granite sport crag about 12 miles from Sondrio that bookends the western end of the valley like the head of a giant spade that some mythological colossus has thrust into the forested hillside. It's my favourite sport crag in the area, boasting rock of far superior quality to the slick, polished schist and gneiss at Sassella, Castelvetro or Ponte and enough variety in the type and grade of climbs – friction, overhangs, cracks, crimpy face climbs, dihedrals, chimneys, arêtes, multi-pitch routes – to make it more like an eclectic buffet or potluck compared to the more *table d'hôte* offerings elsewhere.

On the approach to the village, a low cluster of a hundred or so stone-built houses ringed around a domed church in the centre, I realise I've been unwittingly taking advantage of the valley's unwritten 20-kilometre-per-hour buffer on speed limits (50 means 70, 70 means 90). I slow to a crawl to avoid waking the locals with the rumble of my tyres on the rutted, cobbled streets. I park next to the stream that runs through the wood in front of the rock face and splits the town in two, grab my gear, then jog up the narrow alleyway towards the crag, which, it appears, I'll have entirely to myself.

I choose a climb at the bottom, north end of the crag called *I Principi* (The Princes), which uses the same anchor as a slightly harder route to the right called *I Principi Diretta* and another on the left called *Ratatosk*. Its juggy holds make this route one of few at the crag that simplify the awkward logistics of rope-soloing as a leader on the first climb, which requires me to stop every few moves and pull enough rope through the self-belay device to allow me to do the next few moves. After securing the rope to the anchor at the end of the first climb, I'll then be able to climb all three routes easily and safely, not as a leader but as a seconder, i.e. when the rope is already in place and the self-belay device lets me climb the length of the rope without a partner or any risk of falling. The three routes are graded 6a, 6a+ and 6b+ respectively. Although I've climbed all three around 2,000 times each, and none requires great technical ability or presents a particularly stiff challenge in normal times, after two months of quarantine, the thought of spending the next few hours adding to that tally has me giddy.

I knot the two ends of my rope and leave a double bight through which I feed two carabiners to clip onto the lowest two bolts, making sure I equalise the tension in both loops so that the weight of impact will be spread evenly in the event of a fall. Aware that I'm out of practice and that my frenzied, madcap rush to get going might be undermining my usual diligence, I take extra care to ensure I've done everything right, checking the gates are screwed shut on my carabiners and that my knots are solid. I put on my harness and load it up with my PPE for the day – ten quickdraws, a belay device for the descent, a locking carabiner, a daisy chain to tie in at the top and my chalk bag. I put on my helmet and shoes, feed the rope through my self-belay device, clip into the carabiner on my harness, double-check everything, then push off onto the rock.

The first four or five metres are an easy scramble on an 80-degree gradient. Every few moves I stop, grip the two lengths of rope in my teeth, and pull enough through to let me make the next move. The crag is silent but for the satisfying clip every time I place a quickdraw, the steady ditty played by the gear jangling on my harness, and the sound of the village below slowly awakening. I clip the first three bolts without problem, then come to the crux of the route between the third and fourth bolts – a long, thin crack that leads up through an over-hanging roof to a ledge with juggy holds. For shorter climbers, this section of the climb can be tricky, requiring them to plant their hands sideways in the crack, one above the other, while edging their feet up in two-inch increments before making a desperate lunge over the top for a large hold on the ledge. I've done the route so many times that I've figured out a way of skipping the hand swap-overs in the crack by starting off with a high right foot, jamming my left hand as far up the crack as I can reach, then making use of a pebble-sized intermediary hold off to the right at full stretch before reaching over the top. If I fell from here, I would drop three metres in total before the self-belay device arrested the fall, counting the 1.5 metres of slack in the rope and the 1.5 I'd drop below the bolt. To reach

Kieran Cunningham

the bolt above the top of the overhang, however, I have to feed
out another three metres, meaning I'll fall nine metres if I get
my moves wrong. I smear my left sole in a dimple in the rock
to my left then step up, placing the toe of my right foot into an
angular pocket just above my hip. I make a bit of a mess of the
next move, missing the sweet spot on the hold for my left hand
in the crack and fumbling about for the least-slick edge before
finally landing it. I take a deep breath before reaching out to
the intermediary with my right hand, knowing that if I make
a similar mess of this move there's every chance I'll be falling.

I land it. I pinch the nub between my thumb and two fingers and shift my weight across to the right to make the next
move, then push with my right toe and reach over for the jug,
which my hand finds by memory. Now I'm dangling in space
from one hand, but all I need to do is use the jug to pull myself
over the overhang and up high enough to reach the next holds.
First I have to lift my feet. I look down for the footholds –
the left foot a pea-sized nub above my knees and the right a
minute indentation just below my right hip. I almost laugh at
how tiny they appear but know together they'll provide just
enough leverage to haul my body upwards. I hang for a few
seconds to catch my breath, alternating the hand I'm hanging from to shake out the other and give each the chance to
recover the strength needed for the move. I'm committed:
the only way down is to let myself fall nine metres, which is
suboptimal, so the only way is up. I point my right toe into
the first indent and am surprised by how stable it feels, then
bring up my left to the second, quickly shift my hands, then
hook over my right heel. After the heel hook, I drop my left
leg in a 'flag', letting it dangle in space below me to redistribute

278

my weight, then reach up for the two holds that take me to the next bolt. I clip in. With both feet now safely on a large, 10-centimetre ledge, I can relax. Having gone sideways only for, give or take, my past 1,500 climbs, going up feels strangely novel. My forearms are already pumped and the fall factor on every move seems twice as fearful as it had done just over two months ago. The surge of energy is like a second awakening for the day, slapping the last sleepy haze of hyperreality out of my system and centring my attention fully on the present.

Hard work done, the rest of the climb is pure pleasure, zig-zagging upwards through a slightly concave dihedral on long horizontal and diagonal cracks with neat, crimpy handholds, occasional jugs and pronounced lateral side-pulls. The route from here onwards is also slightly overhanging – while more strenuous, it means that any fall will be into space, not onto the rock below.

I'm now about 20 metres above the foot of the crag. I pause every so often to look down and at my surroundings: the dome of the church in the village below; my car, like a blue pebble, parked in the building's shadow; the lush, Neverland-ish forest in front of the crag, to my right; and the swifts darting around the rock above me. Each time I look down, I feel a giddiness I haven't experienced since my first few outings with my father as a child.

While many of the holds are familiar, it feels like I'm discovering much of the route anew. The rock surprises me with its solidity every time I lay my hand on a hold – a nov-elty given the dislodging tendency of the rocks in the Dusk Wall. Though pleased by how much of my finger strength I've retained by training on the garden and house walls, what once felt like mantelpieces, shelves, and jugs now feel like knife blades and thimbles, forcing me to pay more attention to my footwork and the positioning of my body on each move.

Near the top of the route I hear the jangle of hardware and see another solo climber 50 metres or so over to my right, partially hidden by the trees – a heartening sight not just from a legal perspective but as a representation of the sense of community that I've missed almost as much as the act of climbing itself. When I reach the anchor, I feed the rope out with my teeth, clip myself onto the second ring in the anchor with my daisy chain and let out a cry of delight that brings a shout of *'Bravo!'* from the hidden climber. It's my first climb in two months. Stage 1 of my post-quarantine renaissance is underway.

When I'm at the top of the route for the third time, I look down and see a Carabinieri vehicle parked next to mine. The suited officers take a look at my car, slam their doors shut and start up the path towards the crag.

Fuck.

I abseil down, put on my mask and take out my identity card, ready to pay the fine: €206 gone, it seems, but it'll be worth every penny. The officers arrive, liveried and masked, sweating from the short uphill hike to the foot of the crag. Before they speak to me, the shorter and younger of the two says something I don't hear to the other, who then turns towards me.

'Buongiorno,' he says, tiredly. 'Are you climbing alone?'

'Yes.'

'No partner?' His mask is suspended fractionally above his face by his stubble. His discomfort is evident, his nose twitching as he speaks and beads of sweat balling on his temples. The smell of their aftershave and laundered clothes reminds me I have neither washed nor laundered anything I'm wearing for somewhere in the region of a week and I'm sporting a haircut that's become progressively more outlandish and convict-like the more I've tried to tidy it up with remedial snips over the last few days. It's not the look of your average law-abiding citizen. Working in my favour, however, is the knowledge that police here tend to treat climbers with a lighter hand. Once, I'd been unwittingly speeding when returning from a multi-pitch route on the Grigna with Pa. After inspecting my passport, the officer who'd pulled us over promptly forgot his duties, leaned back on the protective barrier, lit a smoke and began quizzing the pair of us about William Wallace, the Loch Ness Monster, Scottish independence, whisky and, oddly, leprechauns, before sending us on our way, fine-free, half an hour later.

'No,' I answer, as the second, taller officer steps to the side for a better view of my set-up.

'But how?'

'I use a self-belay device.' I grab the device from the rope. 'See?'

They exchange a few muffled words, turning their heads so I can't hear.

'Is there a problem?' I ask, while they're still mid-huddle. Their hands are aflutter in that more languorous way that usually translates into a lack of interest or caring, or a sense of futility in the object of discussion. The taller one's raised shoulders, upturned palms and pleading eyes suggest him having reluctantly assumed the role of bad cop for the sake of form (in Italy, no decision, no matter how small, can be taken without a thorough, circuitous verbal measurement of each option's merits); the shorter one's repetition of the ubiquitous four-finger-and-thumb pinch wagging gesture suggests he's on my side and is having none of it.

They turn back to face me, the taller one's scolded-looking eyes settling somewhere high on the crag above me while the shorter of the two delivers the verdict.

'Nah,' says the shorter one with a shrug, a smile showing in the creases of skin around his eyes. 'No problem. Looks like you've found a loophole. Be safe!'

I continue climbing after the Carabinieri leave. Before Istanbul, I was coming here three times a week, doing some twenty-five climbs, mostly wearing a backpack filled with five kilogrammes of weights to increase the difficulty and keep myself in shape throughout the winter. Today, after completing sixteen routes, each of which takes around ten minutes, I'm spent. I pack away my gear slowly, enjoying the breeze, the sunlight filtering through the canopy of the trees, the sheer spaciousness. When I'm done, I sit on a rock at the foot of the crag. The feeling of release is instantaneous and total – like sex after an extended dry spell. But the benefit is far from purely physical. As with any climbing session, it feels as though the time I've spent at the crag has been enclosed within a set of parentheses protected from the clamour and mess of the narrative playing out on either side of it. Now that the mess is worse and the need for reprieve more pressing than ever, its value inflates exponentially. It is not only atonement and compensation for the stresses of the days past but an inoculation against whatever others might transpire in the days ahead. With my main coping tool returned to my armoury, I'm no longer worried about an episode. A few more days like this, I'm sure, and I'll be back on an even keel.

Lockdown Day 60

Staying inside when it's finally possible to go out feels like blasphemy, but I'm pacing myself. Stage 1 of my post-quarantine renaissance is done; Stage 2 will start tomorrow.

I work until three, marvelling all the while at how much easier it is to function now that I've been able to leave the house and clear my head. My body feels as though it's shot with a dose of morphine, my brain like the lid's been lifted to let out the steam. My sleep was more of a mini-coma, lasting a full, uninterrupted eight hours – something that hasn't happened since I left Istanbul.

Internal weather-check: a slight casing of recent inclemencies and unsettledness in the days ahead with a generally brighter picture possibly emerging towards the end of the week (but bring your brolly just in case).

When I'm done with work, I go to the garden to do some stretching on the lawn. While I'm there, I remember that I've neglected the azalea for a few days and head inside to fill the watering can.

When I return to the garden, I see Beatrice, Giuseppina's daughter from Novara, climbing up through the vines from Via Scarpatetti.

'What are you doing?' she asks when she sees me. I've done the watering and now I'm removing the improvised sunshade Giuseppina and I made with a couple of bamboo supports and a rubbish bag. Beatrice is the most similar to Giuseppina of all the three daughters, her hair cut in a near-identical bob and her rosy, sanguine face always seemingly on the cusp of an earnest, ebullient smile.

'Looking after your dad's azalea,' I say. 'The gardener wasn't able to come during the *quarantena* so your mum asked me to look after it – because of her allergy, you know?'

Her face tells me she doesn't know, her brow crumpled with confusion until she lets out a little parp of laughter.

'Kieran, *caro*,' she says, barely able to contain her mirth. 'Those are geraniums.'

I look down at the bush accusingly. It's a pink, bushy affair. Azalea-like, I'm sure.

'Are you sure?'

'Of course I'm sure! I planted this with her about ten years ago. And my dad never set foot in this garden unless it was to lay out his deckchair and drink a beer. He never took any interest in plants whatsoever. You've been had!'

'What? Why would she—?'

'Let's ask her.'

She screams in the direction of the house. The sort of scream that elsewhere would have me scanning the surrounding terrain for imminent avalanches. Giuseppina appears on her terrace, duster in hand, a few moments later.

'Mamma, why did you tell this poor lad that this was an azalea?' Beatrice says, irreverently toeing the bush and causing a few petals to drop onto the grass. 'And that you're allergic?'

'How else was I to get him out of the house? If I didn't, he was just going to sit in front of his computer all day.'

She smiles unapologetically, shrugs, swats at something in the corner of the doorframe with her duster, then returns inside.

I'd always thought Giuseppina's worry consisted of precisely nine elements made up of her three daughters, three sons-in-law and three grandchildren. My accounting was off – to believe there were any fewer than ten parts would be to do her a gross injustice.

Later that evening, while the promised thunderstorm is growling over the valley, Beatrice appears at my door clutching a plastic bag.

'These are for you,' she says, handing me the bag, 'to say thank you. I washed them first. Promise.'

I open the bag. Inside there are five or six masks made with what appear to be bra straps and material from either table-cloths or curtains.

'*Grazie!*' I say, slightly disappointed not to find some of the little pistachio biscuits she sometimes brings me as reward for cutting the grass or driving Giuseppina to her doctor's appointments. 'But thank me for what?'

'For looking after Mamma. She felt much better throughout all this knowing you were there if she needed you.'

'You're welcome,' I say, 'but you do know that she's been the one looking after me, right?'

'*Ma, sei pirla!* [You're daft!] Haven't you understood yet? That's how you look after her – just by giving her something or someone to fret over.'

'I had my suspicions.'

'Anyway, thanks for letting her.'

Aiyla calls me when I'm in bed. Our arguments from last week have been shelved and we keep our conversation on safe ground. She tells me Turkey's about to let kids and over-sixty-fives leave their homes for the first time in weeks, is sending PPE to every nation in the world despite its own medical

staff having to reuse masks and gowns, and is in the middle
of Ramadan. This morning, she had to drive to her office to
collect some documents. While on the motorway between her
university and her parents' home on the Asian side of Istanbul,
she saw a kitten scampering through the traffic. She pulled
onto the hard shoulder, reversed back to where she'd seen the
kitten and spotted it hunkered down between the outside lane
and central reservation, frozen to the spot. When she got out
the car, however, it had disappeared. She drove home in tears,
only to hear a kitten-like squeal from under her car bonnet
once she'd parked at home. When she opened the bonnet,
she found the cat, who's now living in her garden and been
named Şansli (Lucky).

Lockdown Day 62

I wake to my alarm at 4 a.m.

I prepared my rucksack last night before bed, so after a
quick coffee I get dressed and leave the house, closing the door
and gate gently behind me.

I drive through the empty streets of town and cross the
valley floor in the direction of the Orobie. I'd had the usual
difficulty deciding which mountain to climb. The avalanche
forecasts didn't look good, particularly for north-facing slopes
and anything over 3,250 metres, so roughly half of the peaks
on my list were ruled out. After four or five hours debating
the twenty or so options that remained, the decision was
obvious: Pizzo di Rodes, the largest of the eight peaks that
have been staring at me through my living room and bedroom
windows these past two months. The normal route goes up

the north side of the mountain, which I can see is still clad in snow, but on my map yesterday I found what looks like a way to the summit from the south, circling round the back via the Caronno Valley before climbing onto a narrow ridge leading up to the peak.

I've climbed Rodes half a dozen times before and each time has been memorable: it was the first mountain in the valley that I climbed in both winter and summer; the first I climbed on skis; and last year I went up there with Lucia, Alessio, Michele and Simona and spent four hours on the summit waiting for sunset before skiing down in the dark, dodging trees and boulders and 15-metre drops after both Lucia's and my own head torch batteries died almost simultaneously on the descent. At 2,850 metres, it's far from the biggest mountain in the area but is ideal in the circumstances – not so high or challenging that I'll be exposing myself to unnecessary risk, but enough that I'll be able to sate my longings for wildness, build up my fitness and exorcise some of the excessive physiological and intracranial tension that's threatened to derail me over the past week or so.

Dawn is yellowing the sky to the south as I park the car on the Piana di Agneda, a boulder-strewn alpine meadow at around 1,250 metres, just past a small hamlet where a few stunned-looking goats are strolling the dirt streets between a handful of rustic mountain cottages and a crumbling church that overlooks the lower part of the valley.

The path starts out flat before zigzagging up a forested slope towards the Lago di Scais, an emerald-coloured lake set in an amphitheatre of jagged, snow-encrusted peaks. After veering left at the lake's south-eastern tip, the path leads through a short, forested section to another alpine meadow at 1,600 metres before rising steeply to an unmanned mountain hut, Rifugio Mambretti, at 2,000 metres. I hit the first snow just above the meadow. It slows my progress, but I push on, determined to make it to the *rifugio* for sunrise.

The sun still hasn't climbed above the peaks to the east when I arrive at the hut. I sit and wait, enjoying the cool air and views of the thinning curlicues of cloud above a cluster of tall peaks to the south-west and the Vedretta di Pirola glacier, which just thirty years ago extended far into the valley below the *rifugio* but now occupies only the upper portion of a hanging valley more than a kilometre away.

I hear movement above me. I turn and see a family of six or seven Alpine ibex (wild mountain goats with huge recurved horns) crossing the hillside above the *rifugio*. Instead of waiting for sunrise, I set off after them, climbing another 200 vertical metres but maintaining my bearing in the direction of Pizzo di Rodes.

I find the ibex on the edge of a near-vertical cliff, feeding on a south-facing slope where enough snow has melted to expose a 20-metre patch of grass. I move quietly to within 15 metres then plant my rucksack in the snow as a seat and sit watching them, taking photographs, until they depart in unison on some inscrutable signal almost an hour later.

I put on my crampons and continue south, climbing a steep slope on harder snow. The crunch of my crampons is the only sound, barring my breath and the occasional whoop of marmots warning their colony of the intruder in their midst. At 2,400 metres, I arrive in a giant snow-bowl littered with avalanche debris from the slopes of the surrounding peaks.

Ahead of me, a steep, 300-metre slope of around 60 degrees lies before the col, a small notch in the ridge above that I need to reach before following the ridge to the summit, which lies off to the left, roughly a kilometre away as the crow flies. It takes me almost an hour to gain the ridge, and another half-hour to clamber my way over the friable rock to a small balcony just below the top. Around halfway along the ridge, I'm smacked by a jarring dose of perspective. Either side of me, there's a drop of around 250 metres. The rock I'm climbing on is mostly solid, but each hold requires a gentle tug to test stability before committing to a move. Occasional lumps fail the test, coming off in my hand with only the slightest resistance. The climbing isn't difficult, but the three or four seconds of air time that each loose rock enjoys before landing at the base of the cliff behind me offers a very vivid preview of how things might go should I slip – unlike sport climbing, here I have no rope to break my fall if I should make the slightest mistake. And yet I'm calm – more than I have been in two months. There's even humour in the absurdity of doing something so patently dangerous voluntarily, willingly, given the last few months' preoccupation with safety.

The ridge drops a few metres directly below the summit onto a humped, rocky ledge, from where a short, steep scramble up a bank of snow-coated talus leads to the peak.

Normally, when I reach the top of any mountain, personal tradition requires that I let out a long, barbaric yawp – a Whitman-inspired tip of the hat to the wild spirit. Today, however, as I plant my ice axe over the slim cornice and take the final step onto the summit, I let out no yawp but, after catching my breath, stand to survey the scene before me every bit as carefully and quietly as I had the ibex, as if it might disappear with the slightest disturbance.

The sky is clearer than I ever remember it being, bereft of the thin bronze gauze of smog that sometimes hangs over the valley on windless days. A coven of alpine choughs skim below the summit. I count off the surrounding peaks like a roll call of old friends at a long-awaited reunion. To the north-west I can make out the humped outlines of Monte Rosa and Monte Disgrazia, and the spade-like south wall of Pizzo Badile, ahead of me I see the giants of the Bernina Range, to the east the more isolated trio of Monte Cevedale, Gran Zebrù and Monte Adamello. The valley below looks peaceful, at rest, glimmering beneath a faint haze of heat rising off the flanks of the mountainsides. I was right: we should be screaming in the streets; that all this exists – mountains, snow, valleys, towns, cities, people, ibex, the lot – is beyond comprehension, too absurd to fathom, and my time in quarantine has only made the absurdity all the more apparent.

In my eagerness to get out the door this morning I skipped meditation. My early start has given me time to spare, so I kneel down and scoop a few handfuls of snow together to fashion a makeshift cushion, then sit cross-legged, eyes open and aimed over the valley below, determined to absorb and devote as much of my attention to my surroundings as I can as a way of treating the withdrawal symptoms I've suffered these past two months.

I've been sitting for around half an hour when it happens – the thought, that is, that I could end it all now. It comes quietly, without fanfare or emotional charge, a natural consequence of forces I can neither see nor fathom but is just as incongruent to the joy I've felt during this long-overdue reunion with the mountains as my manic exuberance was during Ma's illness. It doesn't rush, doesn't shout, just sidles casually into my mental landscape, obscuring all else from view, as compelling and incontestable as the mountains surrounding me.

The thought is seductive, throwing an elbow and a wink to the lingering suspicion I've always harboured that the life I've built these past six years was bound to come crashing down sooner or later. In my life before Sondrio, this was the thing that sustained me as much as anything – the knowledge that, when it all got to be too much, I could end it. All could be nothing in the blink of an eye. It was the get-out clause to the whole mess. It was my happy thought. It's never happened because each time I've come within hitting distance of the Big D, there's always been conflict, some tug back lifewards – the thought of the anguish I'd cause, heart-rending mental images of the world that would carry on without me, or some rogue strain of optimism that convinced me that it mightn't be so bad, that this last try might be better than any of the other last tries. On other occasions, the thought's allure was emotionally charged and largely devoid of logic. This time, however, its reasoning is just as compelling. The shifting of the goalposts, it tells me, has given me a get-out-of-jail-free card. Before Sondrio, I assumed I'd go through life always marginally on the safe side of existential insolvency, always doing just enough to make living a more attractive option than not living, collecting just enough trinkets of solace and succour and happiness, like stepping stones across a swamp, to sustain me through the struggle and sway the balance in favour of continuance. This is how it is for most of us – we run marathons for the reward of thimblefuls of water along the way.

While much is as yet unknown, it's clear that maintaining this balance will be far trickier in the years ahead, that the new terrain and topography of the post-quarantine world will be less accommodating, less forgiving and provide less margin for error by far. And who knows how much or what other forms of shiteness there might be? While I've always been too well off to the tune of a mother, father, sister and a few good friends for a conscience-free discharge, I've always known that there might come a time when my interests in suffering no longer outweigh theirs in having me stick around. This, my thoughts are telling me, might be it. Could they now, knowing what they know, begrudge me a premature exit? It would go down as an accident – 'Scotsman Perishes in Alps Climbing Fall' – or at the very least be put down to a tragic consequence of the strains of quarantine.

I get to my feet and step over to look down the north-eastern face. Two feet from the front point of my crampons, the summit curves over a cornice before disappearing into space. I shuffle forward another few inches and see the car-sized chunks of avalanche debris and boulders littering the snow slopes some 800 or 900 feet below.

I've been here before, of course. There was the date with Grandad's gun in Ma and Pa's shed; the overdoses; a few airy meditations on clifftops; a lengthy staring match with a crevasse on the Palü Glacier. I've even tried a noose on for size. On each occasion, by this stage I'd be huddled up, knees hugged to my chest, crying as much for the life I would live if I didn't go through with it as that I wouldn't if I did.

This time, I'm calm. All the time I've being standing here I've watched the thoughts come at me, as detached from them as I am the plumes of cloud scudding over the tops of the Retiche and the organ-like buttresses of Pizzo Coca and Punta Scais. They come, engulfing me and obliterating the view, then pass. Rather than scare or consume me, their visit is like a chance encounter with an old acquaintance, a reminder both of how far I've come since we first met and how much I'd have missed had our paths not diverged. I'm going nowhere. The world below me is no scarier than the one I walked into after hearing the word 'Bipolar' for the first time in a one-roomed, woodchip-walled doctor's surgery in Edinburgh as a teenager. Just as time and experience have removed the fuse from the fear that gripped me during my first exposure to heights in a lofty notch between the buttresses of Stob Coire nan Lochan with Pa nearly thirty-five years ago, they've made me better equipped than ever before to deal with whatever awaits me in the coming months. These thoughts will always be there, maybe, but their credibility and persuasiveness ebb with each appearance. If I can survive them in the middle of a pandemic, when nearly everything I've relied upon to stave them off in the past has been reduced to a virtual shell of itself, there's no reason I can't do so each of the next times. Experience is its own antidote. I'll get through whatever's coming, I know now, because I've been getting through all my life.

I retrace the route back to the Mambretti hut. It's not yet 1 p.m. I'd left early to cross the snow while it was still frozen from the night before, but hadn't considered the seven, eight, nine hours I'd spend back in my apartment after returning home so early. I don't want to go home. Not yet.

My favourite mountain in the region, Pizzo Redorta, lies just to the south, another vertical kilometre above the *rifugio* at the end of a narrow, four-kilometre valley shaped like a ship's hull and flanked on both sides by 600-metre walls. Yesterday I excluded it as an option after reading the avalanche forecasts, but from the spot where I watched the ibex I saw that the slopes on either side of the valley have already avalanched and the main gulley appeared stable, with enough snow to provide solid bridges over the crevasses in the Scais glacier but not enough to make the slopes 'loaded' and liable to avalanche, even in the warmth of the afternoon sun.

Before common sense can intervene, I'm on my way. Three and a half hours, a glacier crossing and a 200-metre clamber up a narrow snow chimney in the north face later, I stand on the fluted, snow-covered, 6x4-foot dais of the summit, with one foot in the province of Bergamo and the other in the province of Sondrio.

I spend an hour slumped against the summit cross, letting myself recover in preparation for the long slog off the mountain, gazing at a pristine patch of blue sky framed by my cramponed feet. I'm amazed I made it this far, but already know I'm going to pay for my over-exuberance on the return leg. The number-one rule in mountaineering: don't go up anything you can't get back down again. While I'm sure I'll be able to get back to the car one way or another, the state I'm in now suggests the state I'll be in then won't be pretty. Number-two rule in mountaineering: *l'alpinismo è sofferenza*. Before trying to coax my aching everything into getting me back to my feet and ready for the descent, I fish my phone from my pack to check my messages – something that always feels vaguely sacrilegious in such settings and always comes with a degree of risk, the potential to spoil the remainder of the day by discovering better-ignored summons from the world below. This time, I needn't have worried: the message is from Aiyla, with a collage of photos she's robbed from my Facebook page. There are about fifteen in total: me and Pa on the summit of Pizzo Tresero about four years ago; with Matteo on the Scalino glacier; with David on Luna Nascente in Val di Mello; with the Brooklyn crowd on High Exposure in the Shawangunks; with Luigi and Anders on the Biancograt; with Ma on the Elie Chain Walk; with all the gang from Valtellina on An Teallach last summer; the two of us together, me grinning proudly as Aiyla winces under my arm, clinging on for dear life circa three feet from the ground at the crag in Ballikayalar outside Istanbul. In all of them I look like the happiest man that ever lived and am wearing the same dotty, faintly deranged smile that hasn't left my face since I first felt it sting my cracked lips when I pulled myself onto the summit ridge. The gap between the image of our lives projected by what we put online and reality is always a big one, of course, but I get the point before even scrolling down far enough to see the caption, which reads: *'You mean THIS shit? Love you! Hope you're having fun. x. P.S. I'm in.'*

On the way down, I remember my first forays into the mountains here, when, on more than one occasion, en route to a peak I'd pass a mountain hut or descending hikers and ask how much longer it would take to get there. (In Switzerland they tell you in steps; in Scotland the customary 'no' long' encompasses durations of five minutes to two hours; in the US they inflate estimations for safety if Democrats or lowball to self-exalt if Republicans.)

'Quanto ci si mette ad arrivare in cima?' I'd ask.

'Ci metti quanto ci vuole,' they'd reply: it will take however long it takes.

I've always considered the ability to climb and mountaineer a passport to uncommon experience, to see and do things I never would have had I not learned the skills and gained the experience required to do them with confidence. Now I know, more than ever before, that it's so much more. Mountains are among the last sanctuaries of sanity and decency our world possesses, one of vanishingly few counterweights to the harshness and busyness and unreasonable demands of life in the valleys, towns and cities below. Rather than lament the existence of my illness, I can only feel gratitude that they're the cure. Whatever the months and years ahead might hold, I know that I'll be able to get through it as long as such places are within my reach or, at the very least, will be there waiting for me whenever I can escape from whatever other obstacles or obligations life might throw in my path.

The normality that existed in January may be gone for ever, but I don't need it. All I need is to make sure the components that made my life so liveable here before the quarantine curtain fell are put back in place. And I'm almost there.

Hobbling down the final stretch above the car another four hours later, I feel purged of everything that caused me to edge towards the brink of an episode last week. The fear and nervous energy threatening to derail me have fallen off in increments with each step I've taken. I'm exhausted. My legs are buckling like those of a newborn foal and my knee screams with every unguarded step. But I feel weightless, my head emptied of thought and body gratifyingly beat.

Now, I'm ready to go home.

Less than a minute after closing the apartment door behind me and collapsing into my chair, my doorbell rings.

'You didn't leave a note!' says Giuseppina when I answer, reaching out both her hands and pretending to wring my throat. Her eyes seem two tones brighter than just a few days ago. Her cheeks have more colour. Her smile seems like it might burst from her cheeks.

She's right. In my excitement that morning I'd entirely forgotten, and only realised when I checked my watch around 9 a.m., not long after I'd left the ibex.

'How did it go? Did you enjoy yourself?' she asks.

'Yes,' I say. 'It was . . .' I search for the word that may relay the experience adequately and settle on: *'bellissima.'*

'Then I'm glad.'

She reaches out a hand towards mine before pulling it back, slapping it with the other and giggling to herself for her absentmindedness.

'Not just yet,' she says. Then, 'Come, sit with me a minute and tell me all about it.'

We sit on the steps below the front gate, where she's left a few bags of compost and more begonias earmarked for planting in the days ahead.

I tell her about the ibex, the pollution-free skies above the valley, the marmots, the view from the top of both peaks, the crocuses peppering the bare patches of hillside where the snow has already melted.

'You speak about these places like they're your family,' she says, chuckling to herself. 'When this second wave comes, you can list them on your *autocertificazione*, I'm sure, or at least as those *congiunti* [kin] with whom you have *affetti stabili*.'

'Do you want me to help with the plants tomorrow?'

'No, no,' she says. 'The family are coming to visit me, and I'm afraid you're not invited.'

Her face is deadpan.

'Oh, don't worry yourself, *ragazzo*!' She says, interrupting my fret with a slap on my wrist. 'You know, when you first came here, we used to worry about you going up into those places all alone. I used to think it was my duty to convince you to stay in the valley, where you'd be safe. It's what your mother would want, I thought. I'm a mother, too, after all. Now, I understand it's my duty to let you go. It is good for you. I say this only because I see how happy you are. You're a polite lad. If I asked you to come, I know you wouldn't say no.'

'I don't understand.'

'I want you to go climbing, *caro*.'

She leans over and plants a kiss on my head, then turns and starts making her way up the stairs. Before reaching the landing, she stops:

'Just be sure to leave a note, be careful, and come to tell me about it when you're back. *Buonanotte!*'

When she goes back inside, I hobble around the house and up to the Dusk Wall for one last traverse. At the end of the wall, I break off a small chunk of schist from one of the stones and stuff it in my pocket to place beside the smuggled mementoes of El Capitan, Mount Everest, the Matterhorn and Annapurna that I keep in my desk, plant a kiss on one of the protruding lumps of rock, then sit on the grass to watch the moon climb above the Orobie and the fading remains of another day – 9 May 2020 – leak from the sky.

Sixty-two days later, I'm ready to believe we're on our way out.

The past four days have dispelled any misplaced hope I might have had that the world we left behind in early March is one we might return to. It will be different, but already there are signs that it may be one improved. As my neighbour Fausto said, now the virus has forced us all to see the sickness, there's hope that more will be willing to play a part in the creation of a cure. Coronavirus has asked a question, and what happens next will be the answer. I have no comment worth passing on what this new world might have in store in the months and years ahead, nor what we might have done differently. It seems the biggest problems present in the world at this moment in time, a few minutes short of midnight on 9 May 2020, are the result of people like me – elected or otherwise – opining on things of which we have no knowledge and despite an undoubted colouring of our perspective by subliminal fears, prejudices and agendas of which we are unaware. I'll stick to climbing.

I have no clue when I'll see Ma, Pa, my sister, my friends in Brooklyn and Fife, or even Aiyla again, and by that time I'm sure these past two months will serve only as a foreword to the saga that is yet to come, and even that will represent only the net of the gross horror that will be the pandemic's overall impact. The only thing I can say with any certainty is that tomorrow I'll wake up and continue to make the best of things with the resources at my disposal and within the limitations placed by forces outwith my control, consoled and emboldened in the steps I take into whatever world awaits by the knowledge that among those resources and within those limitations there are Giuseppinas, Hollys, Aiylas, Faustos, Enzos, Lucias, Luigis, Micheles, Matteos, Mas, Pas and rocks, crags and mountains aplenty to make the future one worth sticking around for.

EPILOGUE

Just as 4 May was dubbed a 'false reopening', my climb on Pizzo di Rodes and Pizzo Redorta and solo sessions at Sirta turned out to be a false ending. Even while up there, I knew that any new 'normality' would be a half-arsed one without the people who made the old one so special. There's an expression in Italian – *'Tutto a posto?'* – that's one of my favourites, not because it's especially characteristic or mellifluous but because of the difference between what's usually taken to be its English equivalent ('Everything okay?') and its literal meaning ('Everything in its place?'). Since reopening, everything has been okay, but not quite *'a posto'*. The mountains and the crags are where they should be, but everything will only be in its place when everyone I'm used to sharing them with is on and at them with me.

Over the past week, more and more climbers have started appearing at the crag at Sirta, despite sporting activity with non-family members still being banned. Today, I wake too late to squeeze in a session before everyone arrives, so I decide to give myself a change of scenery by climbing at Fusine. The crag there is located in a secluded gorge and its lack of easier routes and the necessity of freezing the shit out of your feet crossing the river between the parking area and the bulk of the routes mean it's one of the least popular in the valley even in normal times, never mind when all the valley's climbers are looking to break themselves back into things gently. In all likelihood, I think, I'll have it to myself.

I *did* have the crag to myself – for all of ten minutes, at which point I hear a yelp from below while fumbling my way up my warm-up route and turn to see Matteo sloshing across the river. His squeal of laughter almost makes me lose my grip on the sloping holds I've been clinging onto for the past three or four minutes, trying without success to figure out the next move. I grab a quickdraw, happy for the excuse to take some of the weight off my already burning calves and forearms, and lower myself off the route rather than risk embarrassment by trying to finish it.

Matteo's drying his feet on the grass at the foot of the crag when I reach the bottom.

'I might have known!' he barks, his voice barely audible over the steady grumble of the river. 'How is it you say in English – "Great minds think the same"?'

His normally coiffed and short-cut red hair hangs like the tendrils of a willow tree over his face and he's for once looking well enough fed that I don't feel the need to force-feed him the energy bars and nuts in my rucksack. He lives in an apartment in a tiny village near Tirano in normal times but during the quarantine has split his time between his parents' place and grandmother's, and the break from his ascetic existence and peanut-butter-sandwich dinners seems to have done him well.

It's the first hugging opportunity I've had since the end of quarantine and, thus, also the first since the last time I saw him, Lucia, Simona, Michele and Co. on 8 March, more than two months ago. Having a real, live, huggable human in front of me wasn't one of the problems I'd anticipated when leaving the house earlier, but the struggle to avoid grabbing him is real. When he has finished drying his feet, we stand for a few seconds, unsure how to proceed. I try to defuse the situation with a curtsey, but he shakes his head.

'No,' he says, 'that won't do. Let's try this.' He turns and angles his backside towards me. 'It's called the *"culo ciao"* – my little cousins taught me.'

I bump my *culo* against his.

'There we go!' he says. 'I don't think it'll catch on, but until we know we won't kill each other, it'll have to do, I suppose . . . What?'

'That didn't really do it for me.'

'Nah,' he says. 'Me neither.'

I have an idea.

'Put your mask on,' I say, pulling on an old fleece. 'I'll wear this, you put on your shirt, and when we're done, we can wipe ourselves down in the river.'

He puts on his shirt and shifts his mask up over his mouth and nose. We stand a metre apart, like a pair of spaghetti western gunslingers awaiting tumbleweed and dramatic suspense music.

'Are we doing this?' I say.

'Kinda feels like you should be buying me dinner first,' says Matteo. 'I've been with my mum and granny the whole time and they've been even huggier than usual. I'm kinda all hugged out.'

'Take one for the team. If Lucia were here, she'd hug me!'

'Okay, but I should warn you,' he says, 'I haven't showered

in a few days. And I did twelve routes here yesterday and spent about two hours at my granny's house cutting the gra—'

I grab him.

It feels good. Almost as good as my first climb back at Sirta and my day on Pizzo di Rodes and Pizzo Redorta; almost as good as the time Giuseppina surprised me with a pat on the head about twenty days into lockdown or when Leigh Griffiths scored twice in three minutes to put Scotland 2–1 ahead against England in 2017.

He stands stiffly in my arms at first, but eventually relaxes into it and slaps his hands on my back.

'Okay, big guy,' he says when I've been holding him for a good few minutes, 'I'm tapping out before you break my ribs.'

I give him once last squeeze then let go.

'Should we climb together?' he asks while we're washing ourselves down in the river.

'I don't know. Can we?'

'Legally, no. Logistically, maybe.'

'Should we try?'

'We've already hugged. Seems like asking if we should try some heavy petting after we've just had sex.'

I climb first.

Throughout the pandemic, one of the recurring themes has been the normalisation of the abnormal and denormalisation of the familiar, something I'm now discovering extends to every aspect of climbing, too: the prospect of taking a flier even just a few feet above the previous bolt is far scarier than it has been since I was a kid; five-millimetre crystals of billion-year-old rock no longer seem ample support for my 85-kilo weight; regaining trust in my shoes' rubber soles to grip glass-smooth, sloping rock is going to be a lengthy process; the ability of unexceptional-looking strands of braided nylon fibres to halt a fall is somewhere between questionable and absurd.

After we've both done four climbs, we take a seat on the rocks by the river to rest.

The crag's one I come to only occasionally, but nevertheless moults memories from every direction. A few years ago, on a slick 6c to our left, I fell while trying to clip onto a bolt near the top and ended up entangled in a tree after pushing myself away from the wall to ensure a clean fall. A few weeks later, David had been clipping into the final bolt on a short 7a+ when he lost his footing and plummeted to within a foot of the ground. The previous summer, I'd belayed him while he'd screamed his way through his first 7c at the crag and beat his fists so hard against the wall in celebration that he couldn't climb for the next week. One day, I think, I'll come back here and remember the time Matteo and I squeezed in a handful of mediocre climbs made momentous by the two-month quarantine that preceded them and an illicit man hug in the middle.

The first message: 'We need to celebrate! La Valle @8?'

The second message: a screenshot of the forecast for tomorrow in Val di Mello – sun all day.

I'd forgotten that 2 June is a national holiday – the *Festa della Repubblica* – and also the first day post-quarantine that interregional travel and *assembramenti* (gatherings) with our friends are allowed. Being a public holiday, everyone will be home and free to climb.

One by one, everyone in the group – Matteo, Michele,

Simona, Lucia, Gaia, Walter, Lello, Cristiano, Leonardo, Sasso – replies in the affirmative.

It's happening.

'Kieran?'

'I'll bring the cigars.'

In the morning, I pick up Giulia in the village of Ardenno and we join the building traffic feeding off the trunk road and heading up to the valley. I met Giulia through Luca a few years ago and we've since become regular climbing partners. We're an unlikely team – she's at least a foot shorter and 30 kilogrammes lighter, but we're well matched ability-wise and together have tag-teamed our way up routes that neither of us could have climbed alone, using Giulia's ability to negotiate delicate slab pitches and mine to haul myself up anything requiring less in the way of technique and more in the way of brute strength.

'Oh, Madonna,' Giulia says, gawping at the train of cars and camper vans below us as we zigzag up the hairpin switchbacks on the other side of the village and into Val Masino. *'C'è il mondo!'* (The world is here!)

The road passes through a series of tunnels in the forested hillside below the village of Filorera before re-emerging into the open expanse of upper Val Masino, where the huge granite walls of Pesgunfi and Monte Piezza on either side frame the towering, sword-like plinth of the Cima del Cavalcorto and the crenellated ring of snowy peaks at the valley's end. To the right, the thumb-like domes of Monte Qualido and Precipizio degli Asteroidi – our destination – come into view, shimmering like giant bronze belvederes in the morning sun. Giulia claps her hands like an enthusiastic seal and drums her feet on the floor. I rock back and forward in my seat, willing my rustic Fiat Panda's puttering engine up the hill.

Outside the village of San Martino, where Val Masino splits into Valle dei Bagni to the north-west and Val di Mello to the east, a dozen or so cars are jostling to get out of the already overflowing car park and the through road is blocked by a throng of tourists wielding ice creams, coffees and camping chairs.

'Don't worry,' says Giulia, sensing my despair. 'They'll be back in the mall by noon.'

A yellow-bibbed attendant waves us through to the overflow parking area on the other side of the village. We find a space and wait for the others.

One by one, while we're sorting our gear, everyone arrives. It's like the first day back at school after the summer holidays. By the time I've been around and hugged everyone, I almost feel like I don't even need to climb; that if we just threw down our packs and spent the rest of the day squatting on one of the rocks around the car park I'd be perfectly happy and the day's mission already accompl—

'*Awwww*,' interrupts Lucia. 'Look who's got all soft and sentimental during quarantine! You really missed us, eh?'

She's right. How much I missed them is only now becoming apparent. All my climbs and hikes these past few weeks have felt like going home to an empty house; now, the house is full.

'Are you nuts?' says Matteo. 'If you stay here, you'll get stampeded.'

The car park continues to fill up as we quickly decide who's climbing what and with whom. We choose to split up to avoid clogging the routes and to meet back when we're done at

Gatto Rosso, the little timber-built restaurant on the walking path through the valley that's become our regular post–climb feeding and decompression point these past few years, and where Cristiano's cousin works as a chef.

I stop and watch while the others rush to prepare their gear and flee the crowds. Lucia's checking Matteo's pack to make sure he's brought enough water and food while he lights up the first of the twenty-pack he'll smoke before we return in the afternoon. Walter and Lello are crouched over the solitary backpack they're taking with them on their climb to save weight, debating how many quickdraws and cams they can reasonably leave out in order to make room for the celebratory beers they're taking for the top. Gaia and Leonardo are having a minor tiff over who's carrying the ropes and gear and was supposed to bring the *bisciöla* (a local fruit loaf). Cristiano, the oldest and most experienced of the bunch, has packed everything in one minute flat and is regaling Sasso with tales of the time his partner was nearly struck by lightning on the Scoglio delle Metamorfosi in 1987 and the time he'd taken a 15-metre whipper after squeezing his hand into a crack and unwittingly grabbing a dozing viper. Giulia's tapping me on the shoulder.

'They're real, I promise,' she says. 'If you stop staring they'll still be there when you look back.'

I stop staring and pull on my rucksack.

'You know the rules,' says Cristiano, when everyone's just about ready. 'Don't die. Don't touch anything that wriggles. If you see anyone dropping litter, throw them in the river. If the Scotsman screams or starts crying, nobody's dead, he's just happy. And if you get caught taking a selfie, you're getting dropped.'

Crying and screaming are on the cards. This place is magical at the best of times, but today everything in it seems like a more dramatic and vibrant version of itself, as if putting on a special show to welcome back its estranged habitués from exile. As we set off, I look around at the others heading up the trail with us – couples, young climbers carrying bouldering mats, families and groups of friends carting up picnic baskets and deckchairs, other parties of climbers with ropes strapped across the top of their packs. Like most climbers and mountain-goers, I usually exult in finding I have my day's stomping ground all to myself, but today I can only exult in knowing that they are here to share the day with us. If every other day since reopening has been about re-establishing the routines necessary to my survival, this one is about *joy*, and the joy exuded by each of them seems to pool with and amplify my own.

My gammy knee and the procession of walkers clogging the main path slow Giulia and me down on the approach. By the time we arrive at the bottom of the route, Lucia and Matteo are already on the second pitch and Walter is halfway up the first, dodging his way around a curious mountain goat who's scuttled across the cliff to see what he's up to and taken a liking to his leg.

We climb quickly but run into difficulty on an exposed, slabby traverse on tiny grains of feldspar crystals on the fourth pitch and an oblique crack on the fifth that's still slick from the overnight rain. At the top of the fifth pitch, we stop to drink some water. We're anchored into a trio of ancient-looking, rusted pitons wedged into a crack in the corner of a giant dihedral, over 1,000 feet above the valley floor. The cliff below us slopes down for 100 feet or so before disappearing from view, ending abruptly. The house-sized boulders, mountain huts and river pools that we passed on the way up now look like specks of marble in the green *terrazzo* of the meadows below.

All the way up, our talk has drifted between the climb and the news that's dominated the headlines these past few days: the killing of two African Americans by the police and white nationalists in the US; the rising infection and death rates in places that chose to rush out of lockdown; the rampant spread of the virus through Africa and South America; the tear-gassing of Black Lives Matter protesters.

As has happened every time I've caught myself enjoying some small happiness these past few days, throughout the climb I've felt unable to enjoy things fully knowing the heartache being endured elsewhere. Like Enzo told me in Giuseppina's garden two months ago, nobody's out of this until we're all out of it, and the events of the past few weeks have shown that 'Out' is still a distant destination.

Yet, as I'm leaning back in my harness in the crack, watching Giulia smiling down serenely on the valley below and listening to the happy sounds of the others above us, I understand my mistake.

This isn't a celebration of the end of the pandemic or quarantine or even the restoration of our freedom. It's a celebration of being *alive*. And the way to celebrate is to live in the fullest way you know. In the town, people will get together in the piazza and drink Aperol spritz and eat pizza; in Brooklyn, they'll cart their dachshund across town in the subway to catch the train to the seaside at Montauk; in Istanbul they'll invite friends round to meet their new colony of cats over a five-course breakfast before going for ice cream along the Bosphorus; in Fife they'll bake a batch of scones and ginger snaps and call on all the neighbours. Here, we climb walls.

The others have flown up the route so quickly that they've decided to throw in an extension over a spooky, overhanging crack on a pitch called *Variante dei Morti Viventi,* kindly leaving a piece of gear in the rock halfway up to help me wriggle through an awkward crux without fear of landing on Giulia's head if I fall.

We find them waiting for us at the top, squatting like a quartet of colourful, grinning, chalk-covered gargoyles on a slim ledge overlooking the entire valley, from its eastern terminus below the crooked hump of Monte Pioda to the wave-like ridge of the Cime della Merdarolla to the west.

Giulia and I huddle onto the ledge beside them and stay there for another hour, passing round a bottle of beer and packets of nuts, watching as the shadows thrown by the ridge of peaks to the south scale the walls below us, slowly extinguishing the twinkling braids of the waterfalls pitching down the mountain's wooded flanks and the flickers from the sun-spangled rocks on the cliffs below.

Giulia and I are last to leave. We reach the bottom of the route in four long abseils and hike down the path to meet the others. The terrace at our usual feeding place is full but by the time we arrive Cristiano's cousin has loaded our friends with plates and a huge bowl of *pizzoccheri* (a local pasta dish), which we cart across the river before spreading out on a grassy clearing by the water's edge.

'You not eating, Scotsman?' Walter asks, when everyone's settled and Matteo's dishing up the food.

'Saving myself for later,' I say. 'I have a date.'

'*What?*' says Lucia, her eyes bulging and fork suspended midway between her plate and her mouth. 'What about Aiyla?'

'I have her blessing, I promise.'

'Be safe, *ragazzo*,' says Cristiano. 'There's more than the clap going around these days. What's the girl like?'

'Absolutely lovely,' I say. 'And wise. And funny. And kind. She was a seamstress, but now she's a keen gardener and full-time caregiver for pretty much anyone who comes near.'

He nods approvingly. 'Nice.'

'And she's ninety.'

'Ah.'

'And her grandson's going to be there too.'

'You're forgiven,' says Lucia, slapping my arm. 'Say hi to Luca.'

No mention's made of the virus. Instead, we talk about how we all got around the exercise ban during quarantine: Matteo hung a fingerboard from his parents' apple tree and jogged back and forth on his grandma's 10-metre stretch of patio; Sasso sneaked out before sunrise twice a week to hike up the hill behind his village in the upper part of the valley; Lucia was in Switzerland for the majority of the lockdown, so was free to do as she pleased; Michele lost three kilos working the vineyard on his own; Simona cycled to and from her hospital job in Switzerland three times a week, each time clocking up 700 metres of ascent over 33 kilometres.

'What about you?' Simona asks. 'You don't look in any worse shape than when this started.'

'I found a new crag,' I tell them. 'I'll take you there one day, as long as you don't mind lizards, scorpions, occasional '90s dance music and the odd vocal spectator.'

Leaning back against a rock, I watch as the others begin recounting the tales of their climbs, doling out the last of their packed lunches for dessert, and laugh and chat and joke with tourists and other climbers passing on the path behind us. I sit quietly, taking it all in, carefully etching every detail into the plates of memory: 'The Day We Got to Go Climbing Again'. A few minutes later, Lucia scoots over beside me.

'You've got that nutty grin on your face again,' she says, leaning back against the rock and nudging me with her elbow. '*Tutto a posto?*'

'*Si,*' I say. '*Tutto a posto.*'

ACKNOWLEDGEMENTS

Especially warm thanks are due to several people: my editor, Frances Jessop, whose guidance and support have been priceless; my agent, Patrick Walsh; Ma, Pa, and my sister, Cathy Cunningham, who are still the largest rocks this side of Everest; Elif; my boss, Brian Connelly; Angela Stringfellow and Ken Lyons; Helen Vernon; Adam Cowlard; Victoria Strickland; Lucia and Michele Battoraro, Simona Pitino, Giulia Mazzoletti, Alessio Poletti, Alessandro Gosatti, Danilo Rebai, Walter Boscacci, David Cassoni, Luigi Branchi, Manuel Giumelli, Laura da Rin, Helios Ciancio, Gaia Perego, Cristiano Rosatti, Leah Rinaldi, Andrew Baker, Joshua Bright, Noah Fowler, Brian Cummings, Samuel Torres, Francesco Spini, Giovanni Bergomi, and Simone Bondio, for being the best climbing buddies a guy could ask for; and, finally, to Clementina, Bruno, Alessandra, Adriana, Paola, Marco, Valerio, Lucio, Danilo, Martina, Camilla, and the people, mountains, and crags of Valtellina, for everything.